Osteochondral Lesions of the Foot and Ankle

Editor

CAMILLA MACCARIO

FOOT AND ANKLE CLINICS

www.foot.theclinics.com

Consulting Editor
CESAR DE CESAR NETTO

June 2024 • Volume 29 • Number 2

ELSEVIER

1600 John F. Kennedy Boulevard • Suite 1800 • Philadelphia, Pennsylvania, 19103-2899

http://www.theclinics.com

FOOT AND ANKLE CLINICS Volume 29, Number 2
June 2024 ISSN 1083-7515, ISBN-978-0-443-13113-4

Editor: Megan Ashdown
Developmental Editor: Anita Chamoli

Foot and Ankle Clinics (ISSN 1083-7515) is published quarterly by Elsevier, Inc., 360 Park Avenue South, New York, NY 10010-1710. Months of issue are March, June, September, and December. Periodicals postage paid at New York, NY, and additional mailing offices. Subscription price per year is $369.00 (US individuals), $100.00 (US students), $397.00 (Canadian individuals), $100.00 (Canadian students), $514.00 (international individuals), and $215.00 (international students). For institutional access pricing please contact Customer Service via the contact information below.To receive student/resident rate, orders must be accompanied by name of affiliated institution, date of term, and the *signature* of program/residency coordinator on institution letterhead. Orders will be billed at individual rate until proof of status is received. Foreign air speed delivery is included in all *Clinics* subscription prices. All prices are subject to change without notice. **POSTMASTER:** Send address changes to *Foot and Ankle Clinics*, Elsevier Health Sciences Division, Subscription Customer Service, 3251 Riverport Lane, Maryland Heights, MO 63043. **Customer Service: 1-800-654-2452 (US and Canada). From outside of the United States and Canada, call 314-447-8871. Fax: 314-447-8029. E-mail: JournalsCustomerService-usa@elsevier.com (for print support); JournalsOnlineSupport-usa@elsevier.com (for online support).**

Reprints. For copies of 100 or more, of articles in this publication, please contact the Commercial Reprints Department, Elsevier Inc., 360 Park Avenue South, New York, NY 10010-1710. Tel.: 212-633-3874; Fax: 212-633-3820; E-mail: reprints@elsevier.com.

Contributors

CONSULTING EDITOR

CESAR DE CESAR NETTO, MD, PhD
Orthopaedic Foot and Ankle Surgeon, Associate Professor, Department of Orthopedic Surgery, Duke University, Durham, North Carolina, USA

EDITOR

CAMILLA MACCARIO, MD
Orthopedic Foot and Ankle Surgeon, "Ortopedia della Caviglia e del Piede", Ankle and Foot Unit, Humanitas San Pio X, Milano, Milan, Italy

AUTHORS

SAMUEL B. ADAMS, MD, FAOA, FAAOS
Director of Foot and Ankle Research, Associate Professor, Department of Orthopaedic Surgery, Duke University Medical Center, Morrisville, North Carolina, USA

AMIETHAB AIYER, MD
Chief of Foot and Ankle, Associate Professor, Department of Orthopedic Surgery, Johns Hopkins University, Baltimore, Maryland, USA

DANIELE ALTOMARE, MD
Assistant Professor, Department of Biomedical Sciences, Humanitas University, Pieve Emanuele, Milan, Italy; Assistant Master, Department of Orthopaedics and Traumatology, IRCCS Humanitas Research Hospital, Rozzano, Milan, Italy

ALBERT T. ANASTASIO, MD
Resident, Division of Foot and Ankle Surgery, Department of Orthopaedic Surgery, Duke University Health System, Durham, North Carolina, USA

AGUSTÍN BARBERO, MD
Ankle and Foot Unit, Humanitas San Pio X, Milano, Milan, Italy

ALLISON L. BODEN, MD
Foot and Ankle Fellow, Department of Orthopedic Surgery, Hospital for Special Surgery, New York, New York, USA

KRISTIAN BUEDTS, MD
Department of Orthopaedics, ZNA Middelheim, Antwerp, Belgium

JARI DAHMEN, MD
Department of Orthopaedic Surgery, Amsterdam Movement Sciences, Amsterdam UMC, Location AMC, University of Amsterdam, Academic Center for Evidence Based Sports Medicine (ACES), Amsterdam Collaboration for Health and Safety in Sports (ACHSS), AMC/VUmc IOC Research Center, Amsterdam, the Netherlands

BERARDO DI MATTEO, MD, PhD
Assistant Professor, Department of Biomedical Sciences, Humanitas University,
Pieve Emanuele, Milan, Italy; Department of Orthopaedics and Traumatology,
IRCCS Humanitas Research Hospital, Rozzano, Milan, Italy; Department of
Traumatology, Orthopaedics and Disaster Surgery, Sechenov University, Moscow,
Russia

BEN EFRIMA, MD
Ankle and Foot Unit, Humanitas San Pio X Hospital, Milan, Italy

ERIC I. FERKEL, MD
Attending Orthopaedic Surgeon, Department of Orthopaedic Surgery, Southern California
Orthopedic Institute, Los Angeles, California, USA

RICHARD D. FERKEL, MD
Attending Orthopaedic Surgeon, Director of Sports Medicine Fellowship, Department of
Orthopaedic Surgery, Southern California Orthopedic Institute; Assistant Clinical
Professor, Department of Orthopaedic Surgery, University of California, Los Angeles,
California, USA

CHRISTOPHER EDWARD GROSS, MD, FAAOS
Professor of Orthopaedic Surgery, Department of Orthopaedics, Medical University of
South Carolina, Charleston, South Carolina, USA

CRISTIAN INDINO, MD
Surgeon, Ankle and Foot Unit, Humanitas San Pio X, Milano, Milan, Italy

JONATHAN KAPLAN, MD
Associate Professor, Department of Orthopedic Surgery, Duke University, Durham, North
Carolina, USA

GINO M.M.J. KERKHOFFS, MD, PhD
Professor, Department of Orthopedic Surgery and Sports Medicine, Amsterdam
Movement Sciences, Amsterdam UMC, Location AMC, University of Amsterdam,
Academic Center for Evidence Based Sports Medicine (ACES), Amsterdam
Collaboration for Health and Safety in Sports (ACHSS), International Olympic
Committee (IOC) Research Center, AMC/VUmc IOC Research Center, Amsterdam,
the Netherlands

JAEYOUNG KIM, MD
Research Fellow, Foot and Ankle Service, Hospital for Special Surgery, New York, New
York, USA

JEFF S. KIMBALL, MD
Orthopedic Sports Medicine Surgeon, Department of Orthopaedic Surgery, Southern
California Orthopedic Institute, Van Nuys, California, USA

ELIZAVETA KON, MD, PhD
Assistant Professor, Department of Biomedical Sciences, Humanitas University,
Pieve Emanuele, Milan, Italy; Professor, Department of Orthopaedics and Traumatology,
IRCCS Humanitas Research Hospital, Rozzano, Milan, Italy; Department of
Traumatology, Orthopaedics and Disaster Surgery, Sechenov University, Moscow,
Russia

WOO-CHUN LEE, MD, PhD
Seoul Foot and Ankle Center, Dubalo Orthopaedic Clinic, Seoul, Republic of Korea

LOEK D. LOOZEN, MD, PhD
Orthopedic Surgeon, Division of Distal Extremities, Department of Orthopaedics, University of British Columbia, Footbridge Clinic for Integrated Orthopaedic Care, Vancouver, British Columbia, Canada

CAMILLA MACCARIO, MD
Orthopedic Foot and Ankle Surgeon, "Ortopedia della Caviglia e del Piede", Ankle and Foot Unit, Humanitas San Pio X, Milano, Milan, Italy

TANIA SZEJNFELD MANN, MD, PhD
Head of the Foot and Ankle Clinic Orthopedic Surgery, Federal University of São Paulo, Escola Paulista de Medicina, Sao Paulo, Brazil

NEIL K. McGROARTY, MD
Orthopedic Surgeon, Department of Orthopaedics, Duke University Hospital, Durham, North Carolina, USA

CAIO NERY, MD, PhD
Associate Professor, Orthopedics and Traumatology, UNIFESP, Federal University of São Paulo, São Paulo, Brazil

ARIEL PALANCA, MD, FAAOS
Orthopaedic Surgeon, Chief of Surgery, Department of Orthopaedics, Palomar Health Medical Group, Poway, California, USA

QUINTEN G.H. RIKKEN, BSc
Student, Department of Orthopedic Surgery and Sports Medicine, Amsterdam Movement Sciences, Amsterdam UMC, Location AMC, University of Amsterdam, Academic Center for Evidence Based Sports Medicine (ACES), Amsterdam UMC, Amsterdam Collaboration for Health and Safety in Sports (ACHSS), International Olympic Committee (IOC) Research Center, Amsterdam UMC, Amsterdam, the Netherlands

SJOERD A.S. STUFKENS, MD, PhD
Department of Orthopaedic Surgery, Amsterdam Movement Sciences, Amsterdam UMC, Location AMC, University of Amsterdam, Academic Center for Evidence Based Sports Medicine (ACES, Amsterdam Collaboration for Health and Safety in Sports (ACHSS), AMC/VUmc IOC Research Center, Amsterdam, the Netherlands

YUHAN TAN, MD
Department of Orthopaedics, ZNA Middelheim, Antwerp, Belgium; Department of Orthopaedics, University Hospital Brussels, Jette, Belgium

FEDERICO GIUSEPPE USUELLI, MD
Ankle and Foot Unit, Humanitas San Pio X Hospital, Milan, Italy

NIEK VAN DIJK, MD, PhD
Professor (Emeritus), University of Amsterdam, Department of Orthopedic Surgery, Amsterdam UMC location AMC, Amsterdam, the Netherlands; Head of Ankle Unit, FIFA Medical Centre of Excellence Ripoll-DePrado Sport Clinic, Madrid, Spain; Head of Ankle Unit, FIFA Medical Centre of Excellence Clínica do Dragão, Porto, Portugal; Casa di Cura, San Rossore, Pisa, Italy

ANDREA N. VELJKOVIC, MD, FRCSC, MPH, BCOMM
Fellowship Director, Adult Foot and Ankle, Division of Distal Extremities, Department of Orthopaedics, University of British Columbia, Footbridge Clinic for Integrated Orthopaedic Care, Vancouver, British Columbia, Canada

COLLEEN M. WIXTED, MBA
Duke University School of Medicine, Durham, North Carolina, USA

ALASTAIR S. YOUNGER, MD, FRCSC
Professor, Division of Distal Extremities, Department of Orthopaedics, University of British Columbia, Footbridge Clinic for Integrated Orthopaedic Care, Vancouver, British Columbia, Canada

Contents

> The current concepts thoroughly highlight the ankle cartilage cascade focusing on the different stages and the different etiologic factors that can introduce a patient into the cascade. Moreover, the authors will provide the reader with a comprehensive overview of the types of lesions that may present as symptomatic, asymptomatic, and dangerous for progression into osteoarthritis, and the authors supply the reader with considerations and directions for future clinical implications and scientific endeavors.

> This article reviews the etiology, clinical presentation, classification schemes, and treatment options for osteochondral lesions of the talus. These lesions typically occur after a traumatic injury and are best diagnosed on MRI. Asymptomatic lesions and incidentally found lesions are best treated conservatively; however, acute displaced osteochondral fragments may require surgical treatment. Lesion characteristics may dictate surgical technique. Outcomes following surgical treatment may be impacted by patient age, BMI, and lesion characteristics.

> Osteochondral lesions of the talus (OLTs) are the lesions that affect the articular cartilage and the subchondral bone of the talus. Symptoms develop between 6 and 12 months after the index trauma and are associated with degradation of quality of life. Two-thirds of the lesions (73%) are located on the medial part of the talus, 28% of the lesions are posteromedial, and 31% of the lesions are centromedial. Currently, OLT of up to 100 mm^2 can behave in a more indolent condition, and above that area, the defect tends to transmit more shearing forces to adjacent cartilage and is more symptomatic.

> Although most commonly found in the knee, elbow, and talar dome, osteochondral lesions can also be found in the subtalar joint and can occur due

to either high or low energy trauma. Diagnosis of these lesions in the subtalar joint is typically confirmed with advanced imaging such as computerized tomography and MRI. Although there are a few published case reports, there is otherwise very limited literature on the prevalence, treatment options, prognosis, or outcomes for patients with osteochondral lesions of the subtalar joint, and thus further research is required in this area.

Cartilage lesions to the ankle joint are common and can result in pain and functional limitations. Surgical treatment aims to restore the damaged cartilage's integrity and quality. However, the current evidence for establishing best practices in ankle cartilage repair is characterized by limited quality and a low level of evidence. One of the contributing factors is the lack of standardized preoperative and postoperative assessment methods to evaluate treatment effectiveness and visualize repaired cartilage. This review article seeks to examine the importance of preoperative imaging, classification systems, patient-reported outcome measures, and radiological evaluation techniques for cartilage repair surgeries.

Biological agents like growth factors (ie, platelet rich plasma) and mesenchymal stem cells are rising in popularity among orthopedics. Orthobiologics therapy aims to fill the gap between conventional conservative therapies like hyaluronic acid and surgery, especially for cartilage disease. Ankle cartilage defects are very symptomatic and could lead to a severe decrease of quality of life in patients, because of pain, swelling, and inability to walk without pain. In this scenario, this paper aims to systematically review the current literature available about biological therapies for ankle cartilage.

The treatment of osteochondral lesions of the talus (OLT) remains a topic of debate as no superior treatment has yet been identified. The current consensus is that it is crucial to incorporate lesion and patient characteristics into the treatment algorithm. One such lesion type is the OLT with a fragment, which may benefit from in situ fixation. Fixation preserves the native hyaline cartilage and offers a direct stabilization of the fragment with high-quality subchondral bone repair. This current concepts review describes the evidence-based clinical work-up, indications, surgical techniques, outcomes, and clinical pearls for fixation techniques of OLT from the Amsterdam perspective.

Bone Marrow Stimulation of osteochondral lesions of the talus has been shown to be a successful way to treat cartilage injuries. Newer data suggest that *Bone Marrow Stimulation* is best reserved for osteochondral lesions of the talus Sizes Less Than *107.4 mm²* in area. Additionally, newer smaller and deeper techniques to perform bone marrow stimulation have resulted in less subchondral bone damage, less cancellous compaction, and superior bone marrow access with multiple trabecular access channels. Biologic adjuvants such as platelet-rich plasma (PRP), hyaluronic acid (HA), and bone marrow aspirate concentrate (BMAC) may lead to better functional outcomes when used concomitant to bone marrow stimulation.

 Video content accompanies this article at http://www.foot.theclinics.com.

Osteochondral lesion of the talus (OLT) is a commune cause of chronic ankle pain. Symptomatic lesions require surgical treatment. Currently, lesions with diameter less than 107.4 mm² are treated with bone marrow stimulating technique with notable success rate. However, more extensive lesions show less predictable surgical results. Autologous matrix-induced chondrogenesis has proven to provide satisfactory medium and long-term results on OLTs. In the current review, we describe an all-arthroscopic technique and the Milan-Tel Aviv lesion assessment protocol.

Osteochondral lesions of the talus (OLTs) are the most common cause of chronic deep ankle pain. Joint-preserving surgeries include bone marrow stimulating, chondral transporting, and cellular-based procedures. Each procedure has its advantages and disadvantages. For that reason, a focal metallic inlay was developed as a bridge between biologics and conventional joint arthroplasty. Despite promising initial results, prefabricated implants are associated with unpredictable results. This article describes a novel customized patient-specific metal inlay as a treatment option for OLTs.

The majority of patients with an osteochondral lesion of the talus (OLT) report a history of trauma. Therefore, it is important to assess for concomitant ankle instability when dealing with patients with a symptomatic OLT. The History; Alignment; Ligaments; Others "(HALO)" approach can be a helpful tool in the evaluation of patients with an OLT. If conservative treatment fails, surgery may be indicated. Although there is a lack of comparative studies investigating the effect of stabilization procedures on cartilage repair, we believe that addressing instability is a key factor in improving patient outcome.

Malalignment of the lower limb, distal tibia, foot, and hindfoot can all contribute to altered biomechanics in the ankle joint, resulting in increased focal pressure. The development of some osteochondral lesions of the ankle joint may share a similar pathophysiology, where eccentric loading to the talus or tibia within the ankle joint can lead to cartilage injury or adaptive changes. While the association between malalignment and the development of osteochondral lesions of the ankle joint may seem intuitive, the impact of realignment procedures on these lesions and patient symptoms remains a relatively underexplored topic in the literature. A comprehensive understanding of the potential role of realignment surgery in managing osteochondral lesions of the talus and tibia is crucial for advancing our knowledge of this challenging pathologic condition.

Osteochondral lesions of the talus are being recognized as an increasingly common injury. Large osteochondral lesions have significant biomechanical consequences and often require resurfacing with both boney and cartilaginous graft. The current treatment options include osteochondral autograft transfer, mosaicplasty, autologous chondrocyte implantation, or osteochondral allograft transplantation. Allograft procedures have the advantage of no donor site morbidity and ability to match the defect line to line. Careful transportation, storage, and handling of the allograft are critical to success. The failure of nonoperative management, failure of arthroscopic treatment, or large defects are an indication for resurfacing.

The last several decades have brought about substantial development in our understanding of the biomolecular pathways associated with chondral disease and progression to arthritis. Within domains relevant to foot and ankle, genetic modification of stem cells, augmentation of bone marrow stimulation techniques, and improvement on existing scaffolds for delivery of orthobiologic agents hold promise in improving treatment of chondral injuries. This review summarizes novel developments in the understanding of the molecular pathways underlying chondral damage and some of the recent advancements within related therapeutics.

FOOT AND ANKLE CLINICS

RELATED SERIES

Orthopedic Clinics
Clinics in Sports Medicine
Physical Medicine and Rehabilitation Clinics

THE CLINICS ARE NOW AVAILABLE ONLINE!
Access your subscription at:
www.theclinics.com

FOOT AND ANKLE CLINICS

FORTHCOMING ISSUES

September 2024
Updates in Hallux Rigidus
James Albert Nunley, Editor

December 2024
Pathology of the Lesser Toes
Caio Nery, Editor

March 2025
Dealing with Chronic Posttraumatic Foot
and Ankle Deformities
Mohamed Mokhtar, Editor

RECENT ISSUES

March 2024
Updates on Total Ankle Replacement
Mark E. Easley, Editor

December 2023
Innovative Approaches on Cavovarus
Deformity: Thinking Outside of the Box
Alessio Bernasconi, Editor

September 2023
Advanced Imaging of the Foot and Ankle
Jan Fritz, Editor

RELATED SERIES

Orthopedic Clinics
Clinics in Sports Medicine
Physical Medicine and Rehabilitation Clinics

Preface

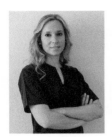

Camilla Maccario, MD
Editor

Cartilage plays a vital role in preserving ankle function, and in general, in preserving movement and a physiologic pattern of gait.

When I was invited to be Guest Editor for this topic, I immediately realized the great opportunity to summarize a decade of controversies and the amazing progress in terms of physiology and pathology understanding, the evolution of imaging and diagnostic tools, and options of treatment.

From a therapeutic perspective, historical treatments have been continuously compared with upcoming technologies. It results in a number of therapeutic opportunities now available in the cartilage treatment "arena." In order to consider this actual scenario as real progress, the challenge for the future will be to collect good data and confirm these new technologies (or at least some of them) as a real step forward.

I believe that in the next 10 years basic science will play a key role in understanding the "ankle cartilage cascade," and also in finding an answer to the simple charismatic questions: "Why do some patients respond better than others to the same treatment?" and "Which key performance indicators (KPIs) are to be investigated?" It will have a tremendous impact on the future, bringing real customization of biological treatments and patients counseling.

It will be a very informative issue with great contributions from some of the leaders in the field.

I would like to personally thank all the contributors for taking the time to share their experience with everyone.

I would also like to thank my mentors, Dr Mark Myerson and Dr Lew Schon, for inspiring and teaching me the importance of learning from sharing knowledge.

Foot Ankle Clin N Am 29 (2024) xv–xvi
https://doi.org/10.1016/j.fcl.2023.11.001
1083-7515/24/© 2023 Published by Elsevier Inc.

foot.theclinics.com

In life, no achievement is accomplished alone, and my final thanks goes to my team-mates (Dr Indino and Dr Usuelli). Teamwork and curiosity feed a youthful mindset, which makes it easy to love my work.

Camilla Maccario, MD
"Ortopedia della Caviglia e del Piede"
Humanitas San Pio X
Via Francesco Nava, 31
Milan, 20159, Italy

E-mail address:
info@camillamaccario.it

Ankle Cartilage
Chondral and Osteochondral Lesions: A Further Dive into the Incidence, Terminology, and the Cartilage Cascade

Jari Dahmen, MD[a,b,c],*, Gino M.M.J. Kerkhoffs, MD, PhD[a,b,c],
Sjoerd A.S. Stufkens, MD, PhD[a,b,c]

KEYWORDS

- Osteochondral lesions • Osteochondral lesion of the talus • Osteochondral defects
- Ankle • Talus

KEY POINTS

- A traumatic injury to the ankle can induce a multidirectional pathophysiological pathway that can induce the patient to go into a cascade of incremental cartilage damage.
- The incidence of (osteo)chondral lesions in traumatic injuries to the ankle is highly underestimated, and every health care worker working together with patients with traumatic ankle injuries should be aware of this.
- Through a comprehensive, active, and multidisciplinary approach, we can effectively address ankle injuries with concomitant cartilage lesions as well as their long-term implications, benefiting both patients and society as a whole.

INTRODUCTION

Osteoarthritis (OA) of the ankle joint is a debilitating condition that significantly affects the quality of life for individuals worldwide. The ankle joint is highly susceptible to injuries, with ankle sprains being the most prevalent among sporting activities.[1,2] Traditionally, ankle sprains were considered relatively benign, lacking long-term consequences. However, emerging evidence over the past 2 decades has challenged

^a Department of Orthopaedic Surgery, Amsterdam Movement Sciences, Amsterdam UMC, Location AMC, University of Amsterdam; ^b Academic Center for Evidence Based Sports Medicine (ACES); ^c Amsterdam Collaboration for Health and Safety in Sports (ACHSS), AMC/VUmc IOC Research Center
* Corresponding author. Department of Orthopaedic Surgery, Amsterdam Movement Sciences, Amsterdam UMC, location AMC, University of Amsterdam, Meibergdreef 9, Amsterdam 1105 AZ, The Netherlands.
E-mail address: j.dahmen@amsterdamumc.nl

Foot Ankle Clin N Am 29 (2024) 185–192
https://doi.org/10.1016/j.fcl.2023.08.009
1083-7515/24/© 2023 Elsevier Inc. All rights reserved.

foot.theclinics.com

this perception, revealing that ankle sprains can lead to substantial harm and contribute to the development of OA.[3,4]

The concept of the "Ankle Cartilage Cascade" has been proposed to elucidate the complex process of cartilage degradation following ankle injuries.[5] This cascade resembles a waterfall, where each stage sets up or "pours down" into the next stage of cartilage damage within the ankle joint and can also be observed and appreciated in the light of a multidirectional pathophysiological mechanism (**Fig. 1**). Understanding the different stages and mechanisms of the ankle cartilage cascade is crucial for identifying opportunities for early detection, as well as developing personalized preventive interventions to mitigate cartilage damage and prevent the progression to end-stage OA.

Underestimated Incidence of Cartilage and Osteochondral Lesions of the Ankle in Traumatic Injuries of the Ankle

One of the critical aspects in addressing ankle injuries and preventing long-term complications is the recognition of the underestimated incidence rates of post-traumatic (osteo)chondral lesions. These lesions can induce cartilage damage and potentially lead to ankle joint OA. Consequently, there is a pressing need to shift the focus toward early detection and primary and secondary individualized preventive interventions, particularly during the subclinical phase of the cascade. Intervening at this early stage may enable the delay or even halt of cartilage damage progression, preventing the subsequent cascade of degeneration and the development of osteochondral lesions (OCLs). The incidence of cartilage and osteochondral lesions have been researched in recent research projects that researched the incidence of these lesions in syndesmotic injuries, ankle fractures as well as chronic lateral ankle instability.[5–8]

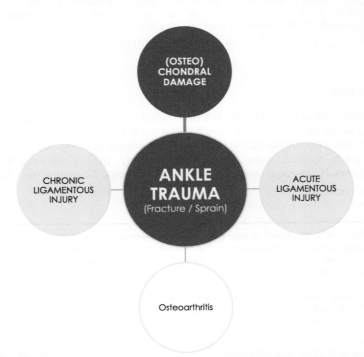

Fig. 1. Seuquential pathophysiological mechanism(s) after an ankle sprain or fracture.

Concerning the syndesmotic lesions, one can observe from the publication by Dahmen and colleagues[6] that the incidence rate of cartilage lesions was around 20%. The study in question aimed to determine and compare the incidence rates of (osteo)chondral lesions in the ankle among patients with acute and chronic isolated syndesmotic injuries. A literature search was conducted, and 9 relevant articles were included in the analysis. The overall incidence rate of (osteo)chondral lesions in isolated syndesmotic injuries was found to be 20.7%. There was no significant difference in the incidence rates between acute and chronic injuries, with rates of 22.0% and 24.1%, respectively. Among the combined group of acute and chronic injuries, 95.4% of the lesions were located on the talar dome, while 4.5% were located on the distal tibia. The size of the (osteo)chondral lesions was not reported in the studies analyzed. In conclusion, this meta-analysis indicates that (osteo)chondral lesions are present in approximately 21% of patients with isolated syndesmotic injuries. The incidence rates were similar for acute and chronic injuries, and the majority of lesions were located on the talar dome. The study highlights the importance of considering these lesions in the assessment and management of syndesmotic injuries in the ankle.

Concerning the incidence of cartilage lesions in ankle fractures, a study by Martijn and colleagues[7] was considered here for discussion. This study aimed to determine the incidence and location of OCLs following ankle fractures and their association with fracture types. A literature search was conducted, and 20 articles with a total of 1707 ankle fractures were included. The incidence of OCLs in ankle fractures assessed immediately after the trauma was found to be 45%. The most common location for OCLs following ankle fractures was the talus, accounting for 43% of all OCLs. There was a higher incidence of OCLs in rotational type fractures. The study emphasizes the clinical relevance of identifying and addressing OCLs during surgical treatment of ankle fractures to improve outcomes. In conclusion, OCLs were frequently observed in patients with ankle fractures, both immediately after the trauma and at least 12 months later, with incidence rates ranging from 45% to 47%, respectively. The talus is the most common location for post-traumatic OCLs. The findings highlight the importance of surgeons being aware of these concomitant injuries and addressing them during the initial surgery, which can potentially lead to improved clinical outcomes.

Concerning the occurrence of cartilage and/or osteochondral lesions in acute lateral ankle sprains, it must be stated that the literature is relatively sparse on this. Whenever aiming to assess the content and depth of the literature, the study by Roemer and colleagues,[9] must be highlighted in light of this discussion. The investigators included in their third Appendix the information that patients with a low-grade anterior talo-fibular ligament (ATFL) injury were associated with the presence of an acute osteochondral or chondral lesion in 17% of the cases. Additionally, in patients with a complete ATFL tear without the presence of any other ligamentous injuries, this rate was 9%. Furthermore, patients with a complete ATFL tear and a partial/complete calcaneo-fibular ligament tear with any damage to the posterior talo-fibular ligament had an (osteo)chondral lesion incidence rate of 6%. Another study that could be mentioned in this area is the one by Taga and colleagues.[10] The investigators stated that 89% of the patients in the acute injury group (acute ATFL injury) had some form of chondral damage. It was found that medial lesions were found in 89% of the patients. It should be noted here that the investigators stated that a poor correlation between the grade of chondral lesions and the extent of the ligamentous injury was found in this acute group.

The last article to be discussed on the incidence of cartilage and osteochondral lesions of the ankle related to chronic lateral ankle instability is also a meta-analysis by Wijnhoud and colleagues.[8] The systematic review and meta-analysis aimed to determine the incidence of (osteo)chondral lesions [(O)CLs] in patients with chronic lateral ankle instability (CLAI). Twelve studies comprising 2145 patients and 2170 ankles with CLAI were included in the analysis. The pooled incidence of (O)CLs in ankles with CLAI was found to be 32.2%. Among these lesions, 43% were chondral and 57% were osteochondral. The majority of (O)CLs (85%) were located on the talus, with 68% of talar lesions being situated on the medial dome and 32% on the lateral side. These findings—besides the other 2 presented studies as above—highlight the significance of (O)CLs in ankles with CLAI, with a substantial proportion (up to 32%) of patients exhibiting these lesions. The talus is the most common location for (O)CLs, predominantly on the medial side. These results can assist physicians in recognizing and treating ankle (O)CLs at an early stage in the management of CLAI.

Toward the Description of the Ankle Cartilage Cascade

Having summarized the under-observed and underrepresented incidence of the cartilage lesions as described earlier, including the impact of end-stage OA extends beyond the individual (as it imposes a substantial burden on society), one can state that it becomes paramount to develop novel and sophisticated imaging tools that can facilitate early diagnosis, as well as innovations aimed at providing joint cushioning to optimize treatment outcomes during the early subclinical phase. By presenting the concept of the ankle cartilage cascade, the authors aim to inspire and encourage further research in the field, with a specific focus on the subclinical phase following ankle trauma. The ultimate goal is to interrupt the ongoing cascade at this phase and work toward the prevention of end-stage ankle OA. Through a comprehensive understanding of the ankle cartilage cascade and concerted efforts in research and innovation, the authors hope to improve patient outcomes, reduce the burden of ankle injuries and OA, and enhance the overall quality of life for individuals affected by these conditions.

In the subsequent sections of this article, the authors will delve into the terminology of cartilage and osteochondral lesions of the ankle as well as the various stages of the ankle cartilage cascade, examining the pathophysiological pathways that contribute to cartilage damage and the subsequent development of ankle joint OA. The authors will also explore the implications of early detection and personalized preventive interventions, as well as the significance of novel imaging tools and joint cushioning innovations in addressing ankle injuries and minimizing the impact of end-stage OA. By synthesizing current knowledge and identifying research gaps, the authors strive to pave the way for future advancements in ankle injury management and the prevention of ankle joint degeneration. By comprehending the terminology and sequential stages of cartilage degradation, we can identify opportunities for early detection and implement personalized preventive interventions.

Terminology

Concerning the manner how one can accurately describe cartilage and osteochondral lesions of the ankle, one can refer to the following article: The article titled "Consensus on the Definitions and Terminology for Ankle Lesions and Associated Features: Results of the International Society for Cartilage Repair of the Ankle (ISCRA) Delphi Consensus" presents the findings of a consensus group that aimed to establish standardized definitions, terminologies, and classifications for ankle lesions and associated features.[11] The study involved 11 questions and consensus statements, with participants providing their agreement or disagreement on each item. The consensus group achieved unanimous or strong consensus on several key points. They defined isolated osseous lesions as bony/subchondral defects without cartilaginous/chondral injury and proposed the term "subchondral bone lesion" for this condition. Isolated chondral lesions were defined as cartilaginous defects without involvement of the sub-chondral bone, and the term "chondral lesion" was agreed upon. For combined osseous and chondral lesions, the consensus term was "osteochondral lesion of the talus". In summary, the article highlights the consensus reached by an international group on defining and classifying ankle lesions and associated features. The estab-lishment of standardized terminology and definitions can enhance communication and promote consistent research practices in the field of ankle cartilage repair.

Different Stages and Etiologic Considerations

From the terminology onto the different stages that are currently part of the cartilage cascade, the authors will now delve into these different stages and into the different etiologic aspects that are part of this cascade.

Asymptomatic Superficial Cartilage Lesions

Traumatic events, such as ankle sprains or fractures, can lead to asymptomatic carti-lage lesions in the ankle without damage to the subchondral bone plate.[12] These microscopic cartilage lesions have historically been considered inert and unlikely to progress into OCLs or end-stage OAand have been referred to as inert in that sense.[13–15] Studies have indicated that the reported incidence of osteochondral dam-age after ankle sprains or fractures is relatively high; however, the proportion leading to poor clinical outcomes remains relatively unknown.[6,7,16,17] Patient-reported mid-term to long-term outcomes following ankle trauma have also been positive.[18–22] However, it is essential to acknowledge that these superficial lesions may contain microscopic cracks, potentially initiating the cartilage cascade, as described by the study of Blom and colleagues.[12]

Post-traumatic Cartilage Cracks with Subchondral Bone Damage and Chondrocyte Apoptosis

Following a traumatic event, cartilage cracks can progress into the subchondral bone, inducing a potential bleeding reaction. At this stage, the lesion may either heal or fail to heal.[13–15,23–25] The insufficient repair response can trigger a cascade of events, result-ing in an OCL and, in severe cases, localized or whole-joint end-stage OA.[26–28] The factors influencing the healing or non-healing of these lesions remain a compelling area of research with many unanswered questions that should be resolved in the com-ing decades. Chondrocyte apoptosis,[29] observed in cases of intra-articular fractures, has also been implicated in the incremental cartilage damage seen in the ankle carti-lage cascade.[30] Biomechanical changes have been observed following impact loads, suggesting alterations in the composition and balance of joint components.[12]

Large Superficial or Erosive Cartilage Lesions

An underlying biomechanical problem or acute trauma can lead to large superficial or chronic erosive cartilage lesions around the ankle. Malalignment, malunion after frac-tures, and chronic ligament laxity contribute to altered pressure distribution, edge-loading, and chronic erosion of the cartilage.[31] These factors result in deep cartilage lesions and subsequent subchondral plate damage. Repair responses to large lesions are often insufficient, leading to scar tissue and fibrocartilage formation.[32] Over time, these lesions can progress, ultimately causing degenerative changes in the entire joint. This process differs from the previous stages of the cascade in terms of its delayed mechanism, with symptoms potentially becoming disabling after decades.[33]

Chondrolysis After Intrasynovial Hemorrhage

Chondrolysis is a separate entity within the ankle cartilage cascade, primarily occurring after repeated intrasynovial hemorrhage or intra-articular bleeding. Mechanical injuries, such as ligament injury/laxity or capsular tears, or conditions like hemophilia can trigger hemorrhages within the joint. These hemorrhages lead to alterations in the cartilage matrix, resulting in superficial and deep erosions and reduced proteoglycan concentration, as well as depressed synthetic activity of chondrocytes.[34] Chondrolysis can progress to subchondral bone damage and joint degradation.[13,14] Chronic ligament laxity may contribute to this process, and intra-articular bleeding can hinder the healing of deep lesions, maintaining chronic synovitis.[8,35]

Implications and Future Directions

Recognizing the ankle cartilage cascade unveils different pathophysiological pathways leading to cartilage damage and potentially resulting in ankle OA.[5] Therefore, emphasis should be placed on early detection and personalized primary and secondary preventive interventions during the subclinical phase, which represents the earliest stage of the cascade. By intervening at this stage, it becomes possible to delay or halt the progression of cartilage cracks and subsequent degeneration, ultimately preventing the development of OCLs and end-stage OA. Achieving these goals requires the development of novel and advanced imaging tools, along with innovations to provide joint cushioning, facilitating the early diagnosis and treatment of cartilage damage during the subclinical phase. By presenting the ankle cartilage cascade, the authors aim to inspire future research focusing on the subclinical phase after ankle trauma, with the ultimate goal of halting the cascade and preventing end-stage ankle OA.

SUMMARY

Understanding the complexities of the ankle cartilage cascade sheds light on the pathophysiological progression of ankle injuries, particularly the development of cartilage damage. By recognizing the sequential stages and underlying mechanisms, health care professionals and researchers can strive for early detection, personalized interventions, and the prevention of end-stage ankle OA. Continued research in this field, supported by advancements in imaging techniques and treatment modalities, will contribute to improved outcomes and a comprehensive understanding of ankle joint health. Through this comprehensive approach, we can effectively address ankle injuries and their long-term implications, benefiting both patients and society as a whole.

DISCLOSURE

No authors reported receiving funding for this study or have any other conflict of interest.

REFERENCES

1. Vuurberg G, Hoorntje A, Wink LM, et al. Diagnosis, treatment and prevention of ankle sprains: update of an evidence-based clinical guideline. Br J Sports Med 2018;52:956.
2. Ekstrand J, Krutsch W, Spreco A, et al. Time before return to play for the most common injuries in professional football: a 16-year follow-up of the UEFA Elite Club Injury Study. Br J Sports Med 2020;54:421–6.
3. Kerkhoffs G, Karlsson J. Osteochondral lesions of the talus. Knee Surg Sports Traumatol Arthrosc 2019;27:2719–20.

4. Kerkhoffs GM, Kennedy JG, Calder JD, et al. There is no simple lateral ankle sprain. Knee Surg Sports Traumatol Arthrosc 2016;24:941–3.

5. Dahmen J, Karlsson J, Stufkens SAS, et al. The ankle cartilage cascade: incremental cartilage damage in the ankle joint. Knee Surg Sports Traumatol Arthrosc 2021;29:3503–7.

6. Dahmen J, Jaddi S, Hagemeijer NC, et al. Incidence of (Osteo)Chondral Lesions of the Ankle in Isolated Syndesmotic Injuries: A Systematic Review and Meta-Analysis. Cartilage 2022;13. 19476035221102569.

7. Martijn HA, Lambers KTA, Dahmen J, et al. High incidence of (osteo)chondral lesions in ankle fractures. Knee Surg Sports Traumatol Arthrosc 2021;29:1523–34.

8. Wijnhoud EJ, Rikken QGH, Dahmen J, et al. One in Three Patients With Chronic Lateral Ankle Instability Has a Cartilage Lesion. Am J Sports Med 2022. 3635465221084365.

9. Roemer FW, Jomaah N, Niu J, et al. Ligamentous Injuries and the Risk of Associated Tissue Damage in Acute Ankle Sprains in Athletes: A Cross-sectional MRI Study. Am J Sports Med 2014;42:1549–57.

10. Taga I, Shino K, Inoue M, et al. Articular cartilage lesions in ankles with lateral ligament injury. An arthroscopic study. Am J Sports Med 1993;21:120–6 [discussion: 126-127].

11. Murawski CD, Jamal MS, Hurley ET, et al. Terminology for osteochondral lesions of the ankle: proceedings of the International Consensus Meeting on Cartilage Repair of the Ankle. J isakos 2022;7:62–6.

12. Blom RP, Mol D, van Ruijven LJ, et al. A Single Axial Impact Load Causes Articular Damage That Is Not Visible with Micro-Computed Tomography: An Ex Vivo Study on Caprine Tibiotalar Joints. Cartilage 2021;13:1490s–500s.

13. Mankin HJ. The reaction of articular cartilage to injury and osteoarthritis (first of two parts). N Engl J Med 1974;291:1285–92.

14. Mankin HJ. The reaction of articular cartilage to injury and osteoarthritis (second of two parts). N Engl J Med 1974;291:1335–40.

15. Mankin HJ. The response of articular cartilage to mechanical injury. J Bone Joint Surg Am 1982;64:460–6.

16. D'Hooghe P, Grassi A, Alkhelaifi K, et al. Return to play after surgery for isolated unstable syndesmotic ankle injuries (West Point grade IIB and III) in 110 male professional football players: a retrospective cohort study. Br J Sports Med 2020;54:1168–73.

17. Rellensmann K, Behzadi C, Usseglio J, et al. Acute, isolated and unstable syndesmotic injuries are frequently associated with intra-articular pathologies. Knee Surg Sports Traumatol Arthrosc 2021;29:1516–22.

18. Gilley J, Bell R, Lima M, et al. Prospective Patient Reported Outcomes (PRO) Study Assessing Outcomes of Surgically Managed Ankle Fractures. Foot Ankle Int 2020;41:206–10.

19. Verhage SM, Schipper IB, Hoogendoorn JM. Long-term functional and radiographic outcomes in 243 operated ankle fractures. J Foot Ankle Res 2015;8:45.

20. Gribble PA, Bleakley CM, Caulfield BM, et al. Evidence review for the 2016 International Ankle Consortium consensus statement on the prevalence, impact and long-term consequences of lateral ankle sprains. Br J Sports Med 2016;50: 1496–505.

21. Yañez Arauz JM. Minimally invasive treatment of AO B ankle fractures: Surgical technique and long-term outcomes. Foot Ankle Surg 2021;27:742–9.

22. van Diepen PR, Dahmen J, Altink JN, et al. Location Distribution of 2,087 Osteochondral Lesions of the Talus. Cartilage 2021;13:1344s–53s.

23. Campbell CJ. The healing of cartilage defects. Clin Orthop Relat Res 1969;64: 45–63.
24. Fuller JA, Ghadially FN. Ultrastructural observations on surgically produced partial-thickness defects in articular cartilage. Clin Orthop Relat Res 1972;86: 193–205.
25. Meachim G, Roberts C. Repair of the joint surface from subarticular tissue in the rabbit knee. J Anat 1971;109:317–27.
26. Delco ML, Kennedy JG, Bonassar LJ, et al. Post-traumatic osteoarthritis of the ankle: A distinct clinical entity requiring new research approaches. J Orthop Res 2017;35:440–53.
27. Saltzman CL, Salamon ML, Blanchard GM, et al. Epidemiology of ankle arthritis: report of a consecutive series of 639 patients from a tertiary orthopaedic center. Iowa Orthop J 2005;25:44–6.
28. Stufkens SA, Knupp M, Horisberger M, et al. Cartilage lesions and the development of osteoarthritis after internal fixation of ankle fractures: a prospective study. J Bone Joint Surg Am 2010;92:279–86.
29. Kim HT, Lo MY, Pillarisetty R. Chondrocyte apoptosis following intraarticular fracture in humans. Osteoarthritis Cartilage 2002;10:747–9.
30. Anderson DD, Marsh JL, Brown TD. The pathomechanical etiology of post-traumatic osteoarthritis following intraarticular fractures. Iowa Orthop J 2011; 31:1–20.
31. Kim J, Rajan L, Gagne O, et al. Realignment Surgery for Failed Osteochondral Autologous Transplantation in Osteochondral Lesions of the Talus Associated With Malalignment. Foot Ankle Spec 2023. https://doi.org/10.1177/ 19386400231163030.
32. Ramponi L, Yasui Y, Murawski CD, et al. Lesion Size Is a Predictor of Clinical Outcomes After Bone Marrow Stimulation for Osteochondral Lesions of the Talus: A Systematic Review. Am J Sports Med 2017;45:1698–705.
33. Valderrabano V, Hintermann B, Horisberger M, et al. Ligamentous posttraumatic ankle osteoarthritis. Am J Sports Med 2006;34:612–20.
34. Wolf CR, Mankin HJ. The effect of experimental hemarthrosis on articular cartilage of rabbit knee joints. J Bone Joint Surg Am 1965;47:1203–10.
35. Hu Y, Tao H, Qiao Y, et al. Evaluation of the Talar Cartilage in Chronic Lateral Ankle Instability with Lateral Ligament Injury Using Biochemical T2* Mapping: Correlation with Clinical Symptoms. Acad Radiol 2018;25:1415–21.

Osteochondral Lesions of the Talus

Etiology, Clinical Presentation, Treatment Options, and Outcomes

Albert T. Anastasio, MD[a], Colleen M. Wixted, MBA[b],*,
Neil K. McGroarty, MD[a]

KEYWORDS

- Osteochondral lesion • Talus • Subchondral • OLT • OLT treatment

KEY POINTS

- Osteochondral lesions of the talus (OLTs) most commonly occur following a traumatic insult, most often ankle sprains.
- Four staging systems have been described that classify OLTs based on different imaging modalities.
- Conservative treatment of OLTs is reserved for asymptomatic lesions and lesions found incidentally; surgical treatment is recommended for acute displaced osteochondral fragments and symptomatic lesions after failed conservative treatment.
- There remains room for improvement regarding treatment algorithms for OLTs.

INTRODUCTION

Osteochondral lesions of the talus (OLTs) are a common pathology encountered by foot and ankle surgeons. These lesions often present following traumatic ankle injuries and occur when the subchondral bone plate or overlying cartilage of the talus is disrupted.[1] This differentiates OLTs from an isolated bone bruise, where local hemorrhage and edema surrounds a subchondral osseous fracture.[2] Although some OLTs remain asymptomatic, some patients may experience persistent pain and ankle instability requiring intervention. Possible treatment options, including operative and nonoperative management, have been widely discussed in the literature, with substantial heterogeneity with regard to treatment approaches and resulting patient-reported outcomes (PROs) and joint function metrics.[3–5] The purpose of this article is to review the etiology, clinical presentation, and imaging of OLTs and provide a

[a] Department of Orthopaedics, Duke University Hospital, 200 Trent Drive, Durham, NC 27710, USA; [b] Duke University School of Medicine, 8 Searle Center Drive, Durham, NC 27710, USA
* Corresponding author.
E-mail address: Colleen.wixted@duke.edu

Foot Ankle Clin N Am 29 (2024) 193–211
https://doi.org/10.1016/j.fcl.2023.11.002
1083-7515/24/© 2023 Elsevier Inc. All rights reserved.

foot.theclinics.com

treatment algorithm for their management as well as a review of outcomes following treatment for OLTs.

ETIOLOGY

OLTs most often occur following a traumatic insult. Ankle sprains are the most common instigating injury, with about 50% of patients who sustain an ankle sprain subsequently developing an OLT[6,7] (**Fig. 1**). Ankle fractures can also lead to OLTs, especially for those patients who sustain a concomitant syndesmotic injury, although these patients are less commonly encountered than those presenting with OLT after ankle sprain.[7–9]

More than 2 million ankle sprains occur annually in the United States, of which lateral ankle sprains are the most common with an estimated incidence of 0.93/1000 athlete-exposures, defined as a competition or practice where an athlete is exposed to possible athletic injury.[10,11] The most common mechanism of injury for a lateral ankle sprain occurs through an inverted and adducted foot, where the ligament at highest risk is the anterior talofibular ligament (ATFL), followed by the calcaneofibular ligament (CFL), and the posterior talofibular ligament.[12] As the ligaments fail, the talus can impact the tibial plafond, inducing an insult to the talar articular cartilage. The mechanism of injury can also correlate with the location of a resulting OLT.[13] In a cadaveric study by Berndt and Harty, lateral OLTs were reproduced by an ankle dorsiflexion and inversion injury model, and medial talar dome lesions were reproduced through ankle plantarflexion and inversion.[14] Lateral lesions tend to be shallow and oval from the shearing force on the talar dome, whereas medial lesions are deeper and more ellipse in shape from the axial compressive forces[13] (**Fig. 2**). Regardless of the specific mechanism, any event resulting in deviation from the ligamentous and bony constraints of the talus can result in injury to the talar cartilage lining, with subsequent bone bruising or delamination.[15]

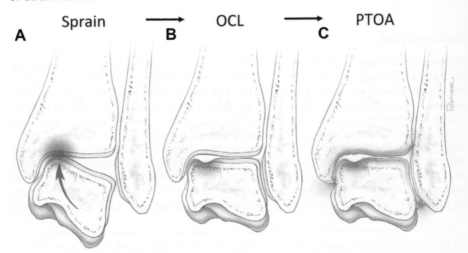

Fig. 1. Post-traumatic osteoarthritis is theorized to progress after a severe ankle sprain. (*A*) A typical inversion ankle sprain results in impaction of the medial aspect of the talar dome on the tibial plafond. (*B*) This impaction injury can lead to the formation of an OLT on the medial talar shoulder. (*C*) The OLT can then progress to posttraumatic osteoarthritis over the subsequent years or decades of follow-up. (Image obtained via creative commons licensing.[111]). OCL, osteochondral lesion; PTOA, posttraumatic osteoarthritis.

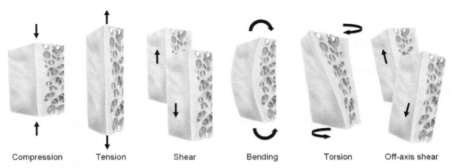

Compression   Tension   Shear   Bending   Torsion   Off-axis shear

Fig. 2. Injuries to the bone and cartilage can occur through a variety of mechanisms, including compression, tension, shear, bending, torsion, and off-axis shear. (Mini N. Pathria, Christine B. Chung, and Donald L. Resnick, Acute and Stress-related Injuries of Bone and Cartilage: Pertinent Anatomy, Basic Biomechanics, and Imaging Perspective. Radiology 2016 280:1, 21-38.)

Less frequently, patients may present with an OLT without any history of trauma. It has been proposed that local ischemia to the bone can lead to necrotic osteochondral fragments; however, it is unclear what specifically results in the ischemia, with possibilities including vascular embolic phenomena or other systemic vasculopathy.[14,16,17] Aside from insults inducing avascular necrosis to the talus, there may be a hereditary component to the development of OLTs. There is a high incidence of monozygotic twins with OLTs in addition to the bilateral presentation of osteochondral defects, occurring in about 10% of cases.[12,18,19] Endocrine and metabolic abnormalities, including hypothyroidism, vitamin D deficiency, and parathyroid abnormalities, may also contribute, with degenerative joint disease and joint malalignment have also playing a role in the etiology of OLTs.[13,17]

CLINICAL PRESENTATION

After an acute ankle injury, pain, swelling, and functional deficits are expected as the ligaments and surrounding soft tissues heal, lasting around 4 to 6 weeks. However, 30% to 50% of patients with ankle sprains experience residual symptoms.[20,21] If after 4 to 6 weeks there remains significant pain, swelling, and limited range of motion (ROM) on examination, an OLT should be suspected. The presence of mechanical symptoms of locking, catching, or clicking may indicate the presence of a displaced fragment. These displaced fragments may lead to the development of synovitis or a large joint effusion. For large, displaced lesions of the anterior talus, the synovitis may be palpable on examination.[22] Other physical examination findings may be subtle, so it is critical to compare the affected ankle to the contralateral side. In some cases, evidence of damage to the cartilage and subchondral bone may only be found arthroscopically. In a series of 31 patients undergoing arthroscopy for persistent pain after an ankle sprain, chondral injuries were present in 89% acute (6–8 weeks) injuries and 95% of chronic (>3 months) injuries.[23] In another series of 30 patients undergoing arthroscopy before ligament stabilization, 67% were found to have cartilage injury.[24] This high incidence was thought to be in part due to injuries resulting from higher velocity impact.

Approximately 40% of patients who sustain lateral ankle sprains develop chronic ankle instability, characterized by decreased ROM, strength, postural control, and altered functional movement patterns.[25] This chronic ligament instability and subsequent microtrauma to the subchondral bone and cartilage can lead to the insidious development of OLTs and should be suspected in patients with this history.[26] For patients that do not report a specific history of ankle injury or instability, chronic OLTs may present as persistent or intermittent deep ankle pain during or after periods of activity. Patients may have normal ROM without any tenderness to palpation or significant swelling.[16]

IMAGING
Radiographs

Radiographs of the foot and ankle are useful for assessing hindfoot and tibial alignment; however, the diagnostic accuracy for OLT is limited, with studies reporting that 28% to 50% of lesions are not visible on radiographs.[27–31] First described by Thompson and Loomer,[31] the heel rise view, which is an anterior posterior (AP) mortise view with a 4 cm heel rise, can double the detection rate of OLTs when compared with standard radiographic views.[28] Furthermore, sequela of ligamentous injuries evident on radiographs including ATFL, CFL, or deltoid avulsion fractures should raise suspicion for OLT.

Computed Tomography

Computed tomography (CT) scans have higher sensitivity and specificity for the diagnosis of OLT at 81% and 99%, respectively.[28,32] CT provides the most accurate assessment of osseous morphology, size, and location of OLTs. A CT scan in full plantar flexion has been found to be a reliable preoperative method to determine the in situ arthroscopic location of OLTs.[33] Although CT lacks the ability to evaluate articular cartilage, this imaging modality provides precise details regarding subchondral bone morphology, such as associated cystic lesions, absorption, sclerosis, and avulsion and/or detachment of a fragment.[34]

Because the integrity of the subchondral bone plate is vital for supporting the overlying articular cartilage, the condition of the subchondral bone is especially critical to evaluate when planning for the optimal treatment modality. In the pathogenesis of OLT, synovial and edematous fluid perforates the fenestrations in the microfractured subchondral bone plate. The continuous high fluid pressures induce osteolysis in the subchondral bone, resulting in an unstable osteochondral fragment and an expanding cystic lesion.[35] Once bone resorption ceases, remodeling occurs and a hypermetabolic state induces dense subchondral bone to form.[36] Nakasa and colleagues reported that the condition of subchondral bone presents on CT imaging correlated with the damage to the articular cartilage and the stability of the lesion classified via arthroscopy.[35] As a final consideration in the imaging of OLT using CT, weight-bearing CT (WBCT) has emerged as a promising adjunct in the evaluation of cartilage injury to the foot and ankle.[37] WBCT allows for assessment of global foot and ankle alignment, which can aid in determination of the utility of adjunctive procedures to collect deformity and malalignment when treating OLT.[38] Moreover, WBCT allows for accurate assessment of joint space width under load, allowing surgeons to more accurately assess progression from osteochondral injury to posttraumatic arthritis.[39]

MRI

MRI yields the highest sensitivity (96%) and specificity (96%) for diagnosis of OLT.[28,32]

Findings on MRI may include the presence of loose bodies, linear subchondral lines extending deep into subchondral bone, cystic lesions with or without bony containment, "kissing" lesions (osteochondral lesions in the same zone on the talus and the tibial plafond), and sclerotic elements. It is valuable when localizing and assessing the morphology of OLTs and can better visualize associated soft tissue injuries and bone marrow edema. However, MRI is most useful in the assessment of articular carti-lage disruption, fragment instability, fractures not identified on CT or plain radio-graphs, and osteonecrosis.[40–44] MRI provides an accurate means of staging (81%–83%) OLTs, although bony edema and thinning of the articular cartilage may overes-timate the severity of the lesion.[44–47] This subsequently impacts treatment decisions because the surgical options for OLT are stage-dependent. Postoperatively, MRI al-lows for the evaluation of bone marrow edema resolution. D'Ambrosi and colleagues importantly demonstrate successful resolution of bone marrow edema as measured on MRI in all but 23.08% of patients with OLT treated with arthroscopic talus autolo-gous matrix-induced chondrogenesis (AMIC) at the 24-month time point.[48] These pa-tients exhibited clinical improvement in functional outcomes. Further investigation may continue to develop our understanding of how pre- and postoperative bone marrow edema grading on MRI impacts surgical decision-making and patient out-comes in OLT.

CLASSIFICATION SCHEMES

Four staging systems have been described that classify OLTs based on differing im-aging modalities. Lesions can be classified radiographically based on the Berndt and Harry[14] staging system: (1) small subchondral compression; (2) partial fragment detachment; (3) complete fragment without displacement; and (4) complete fragment detachment with displacement. Ferkel and colleagues[16] developed a CT-based stag-ing system emphasizing bony morphology and cystic characteristics. Each stage is defined as follows: (I) cystic lesion in talar dome with intact roof; (IIa) cystic lesion with communication to talar dome surface; (IIb) open articular surface lesion with over-lying nondisplaced fragment; (III) nondisplaced lesion with lucency; and (IV) displaced fragment. Hepple[27] devised a system based on MRI findings: (1) articular cartilage damage only; (2a) cartilage injury with underlying fracture and surrounding bony edema; (2b) cartilage injury with underlying fracture without surrounding bony edema; (3) detached but nondisplaced fragment; (4) displaced fragment; and (5) subchondral cyst formation. Last, Pritsch[49] described an arthroscopic classification scheme based on the condition of the overlying articular cartilage. Each stage is defined as follows: (1) smooth and intact but soft; (2) rough surface; (3) fibrillation/fissures; (4) flap present or bone exposed; (4) loose, nondisplaced fragment; and (5) displaced fragment.

These staging systems are useful to better understand lesion morphology, but no single classification scheme provides evidence-based guidance for surgical treat-ment. Instead, surgeons rely on a combination of weight-bearing radiographs, CT scans, and MRI findings to develop the optimal treatment strategy for each patient. Arthroscopy is the gold standard for assessing the articular surface of the talar dome.

TREATMENT
Conservative Treatment

Conservative treatment of OLT should be pursued for asymptomatic lesions and le-sions found incidentally. Special considerations need to be given to skeletally imma-ture patients, older patients with lower functional status, and patients with osteoarthritis. Asymptomatic lesions should be followed closely, but patients may participate in activities as tolerated. For acute symptomatic nondisplaced OLTs, conservative management consists of immobilization for 4 to 6 weeks, touchdown weight-bearing restrictions, and nonsteroidal anti-inflammatory drugs for pain.[50] Weight-bearing precautions in the acute setting are crucial, as reduced contact pressure on the lesion can prevent the forceful entry of synovial fluid into the developing OLT, limiting further damage to the articular cartilage and subchondral bone.

Surgical Treatment

Surgical treatment is recommended for acute displaced osteochondral fragments and symptomatic lesions after failed conservative treatment.

1. Exposure

Ankle arthroscopy allows for assessment of cartilaginous stability, debridement of OLT lesions, and implementation of bone marrow stimulation (BMS) techniques. A standard arthroscopic approach of the ankle should be performed in the supine position using anteromedial and anterolateral portals. Accessory medial and/or accessory lateral portals may be used to improve visualization. For posterior talar dome lesions inaccessible through anterior ankle arthroscopy, the patient can be positioned prone, which enables the use of posterolateral and posteromedial portals.[51,52] A noninvasive distraction device can be applied to the foot for intermittent distraction if required. A tourniquet may be placed around the upper thigh, but arthroscopy is often performed without insufflation.

For larger lesions and lesions requiring perpendicular access for resurfacing or fixation, standard soft tissue and bony exposures to the ankle should be used. Individual variability may limit or improve access to the talar done depending on bony morphologic characteristics and ligamentous laxity. Patients with increased laxity are less likely to require more invasive approaches such as malleolar osteotomy for lesion exposure. However, when needed for extensive lesions requiring wide visualization, osteotomies substantially increase access to the talar dome. A medial or lateral malleolar osteotomy provides complete access to the retrospective laterality of the talar dome in the sagittal plane.[53] In a cadaver model, this study found that only 15% of the posterocentral talar dome remained inaccessible with combined medial and lateral malleolar osteotomies.[53] Other investigators have argued for a more limited use of osteotomy, asserting that greater than 75% of the talar dome can be accessed without an osteotomy via standard anteromedial, posteromedial, or anterolateral approaches alone.[53]

The biplanar medial malleolar osteotomy technique, as described by Alexander and Watson,[54] provides improved perpendicular access to the medial talar dome and can be easily fixated with two screws.[53] The oblique distal fibular osteotomy requires division of the ATFL for external rotation of the fragment.[53,55,56] An anterolateral (Chaput) osteotomy technique uses a small (1 × 1.5 cm) fragment of the anterior lateral tibial plafond.[57] This osteotomy provides a mean 22% increase in exposure of the anterolateral dome when combined with an anterolateral approach.[53] For medial lesions, a medial malleolar osteotomy provides perpendicular access for osteochondral grating or repair. If the medial lesion requires debridement and BMS only, a posteromedial or anteromedial approach without osteotomy may be used. For lateral lesions, an anterolateral approach will allow for perpendicular access. For larger and central lateral lesions, an anterolateral approach with a small Chaput osteotomy can be used.[53]

2. Symptomatic and stable cartilaginous lesions

When symptomatic lesions are associated with a subchondral cyst but have intact overlying cartilage, treatment with arthroscopy and retrograde drilling can result in excellent outcomes.[56–60] Defects should be assessed for the stability of articular cartilage on MRI and again during diagnostic arthroscopy. Retrograde drilling involves a non-transarticular approach visualized under fluoroscopy. The advantage of retrograde drilling is the ability to drill to the level of subchondral cyst without violating the articular cartilage. This technique debrides the lesion and initiates intraosseous blood vessel disruption (**Figs. 3–5**). This promotes revascularization of subchondral bone and induces new bone formation.

3. Symptomatic and unstable cartilaginous lesion

For symptomatic, unstable cartilaginous lesions (<15 mm in diameter), an appropriate treatment algorithm begins with arthroscopic debridement and excision of unstable damaged cartilage.[61–63] Debridement should extend to a stable rim of cartilage surrounding the lesion. Any loose bodies should be removed and a thorough curettage of underlying necrotic bone and scar tissue down a bleeding bed of subchondral bone should be performed. BMS with microfracture can also be implemented. Perforation of subchondral bone with a microfracture awl or drill allows progenitor cells to fill the lesion and stimulate repair leading to the formation of fibrocartilage.[64]

4. Large symptomatic cartilaginous lesions

For large lesions (>12 mm in diameter) with secondary arthritic changes, an osteochondral autograft transfer technique should be considered. This technique replaces and reconstructs the osteochondral lesion with autologous hyaline cartilage plugs[65–68](**Fig. 6**). Multiple small diameter cylindrical autograft plugs (mosaicplasty) are harvested from the ipsilateral lateral femoral condyle. After the talar lesion is fully debrided as described above, the autologous grafts are implanted into the defect. As detailed above, an open soft tissue approach and/or osteotomy will be required to gain appropriate access to the lesion.

Osteochondral allograft transfer provides an effective alternative to autografts[69](-**Figs. 7–9**). Allografts should be used for large, uncontained talar shoulder and cystic lesions. This technique offers the ability to treat large lesions and has no associated donor-site morbidity. Articular resurfacing with allografts restores the mechanical integrity and surface contour while providing more flexibility to restore defects. The

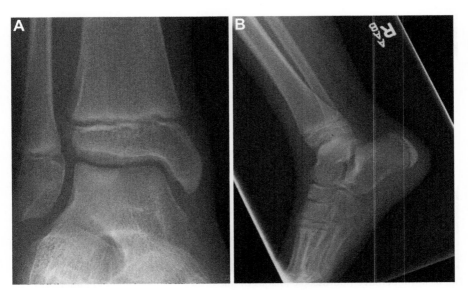

Fig. 3. (*A,B*) Plain radiographs (AP and lateral) of 9-year-old female with a right OLT.

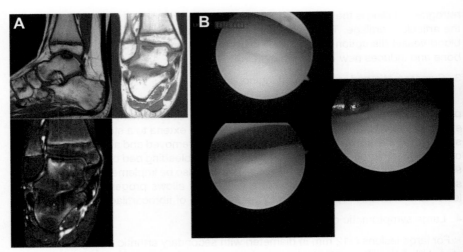

Fig. 4. (*A*) Sagittal and coronal imaging of a 9-year-old female with a right OLT with subchondral enhancement representing bony edema. (*B*) Arthroscopic images reveal an OLT with a stable cartilage cap.

grafts are obtained from human cadavers from licensed tissue patients. Fresh grafts are recommended over fresh-frozen allografts due to chondrocyte viability.[70]

5. Failed debridement and BMS

If arthroscopic debridement and BMS techniques fail to improve symptoms and/or lesion size progresses, cartilage resurfacing techniques such as osteochondral allograft or autograft transfers should be considered. Any associated hindfoot deformities

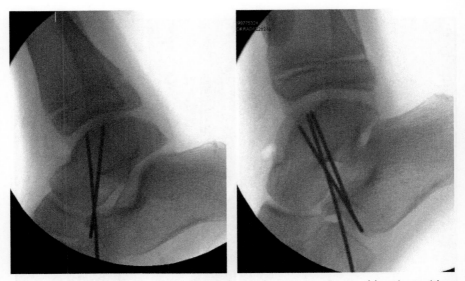

Fig. 5. Intraoperative fluoroscopic images of microfracture in a 9-year-old patient with an OLT with a stable cartilage cap and underlying bone marrow edema confirmed on MRI.

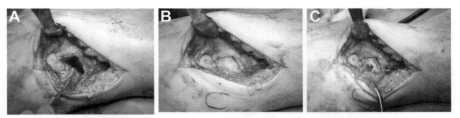

Fig. 6. Osteochondral autograft mosaicplasty using Chaput osteotomy. (*A*) A Chaput osteotomy is made at the level of the tibial plafond to gain access to the OLT. (*B*) After placement of osteochondral autograft mosaicplasty plugs, the Chaput osteotomy is closed. (*C*) The osteotomy is fixated with cannulated screws.

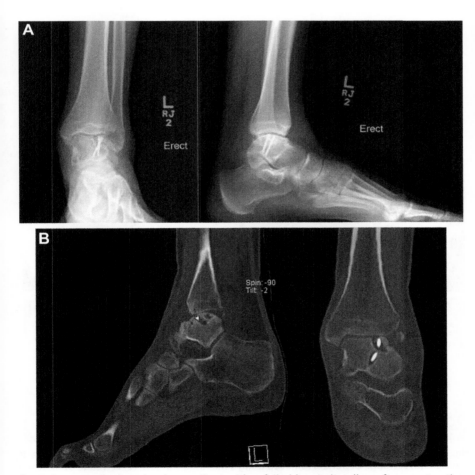

Fig. 7. Preoperative imaging in a patient with a failed hemitalar allograft reconstruction. (*A*) Preoperative AP and lateral imaging of the left ankle revealing subchondral sclerosis and collapse of hemitalar allograft. (*B*) Preoperative sagittal and coronal CT imaging revealing collapse and subchondral cystic change of the previous hemitalar allograft.

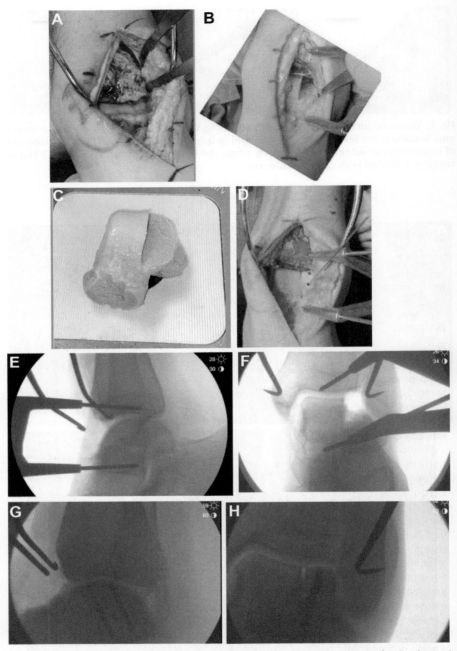

Fig. 8. (*A*) The anterior ankle is approached and the diseased region of talar bone is exposed. (*B*) A wedge of bone is removed using a microsagittal saw. (*C*) A wedge of matched allograft talus is sized and shaped meticulously using the saw to within 1 mm of the articular surface. (*D*) The allograft wedge is fixated in place using two headless compression screws. (*E, F, G,* and *H*) Intraoperative fluoroscopic images demonstrating revision hemitalar reconstruction.

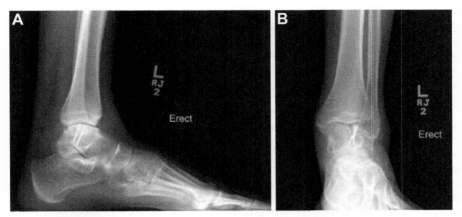

Fig. 9. Postoperative images after revision hemitalar allograft reconstruction. (*A,B*) Lateral and AP imaging revealing graft in excellent positioning with interval healing.

and ligamentous instability should be addressed, as these pathologies may contribute to increased contact pressures on the OLT and failure of conventional treatment options.

DISCUSSION AND OUTCOMES

Perfecting treatment algorithms for OLT, especially in the setting of subchondral involvement, has proved difficult, and multiple reports with conflicting data have been presented over the last several decades. Multiple questions still remain unanswered within the literature, such as which lesions are most likely to go on to lead to chronic ankle pain and the development of osteoarthritis, what are the specific indications for the various treatment options, and which biologic adjuncts show cost-efficacy and clinical superiority when compared with others.

Moreover, it may be inappropriate to use osteochondral injury in other regions of the body as a surrogate for prognosis and treatment options in the ankle. McCollum and colleagues have pointed out that findings of a bone bruise on MRI indicating underlying bone marrow edema are common after anterior cruciate ligament rupture, but that many of the knees involved do not suffer significant chondral loss as a result of the underlying contusion and bone marrow edema resolves relatively quickly.[12] Similar findings have not been observed in the ankle. Sijbrandij and colleagues demonstrate the persistence of edema in the talus for 11 to 12 months on average and up to 17 months after injury with confirmed contusion on serial MRI.[71] However, the clinical ramifications of the delayed healing observed in the ankle remain poorly understood. Some investigators have reported low rates of progression to osteoarthritis at an average follow-up of 6 years for OLTs.[72] Others believe that OLTs, especially in the presence of other concomitant pathologies such as recurrent lateral ligamentous sprain or hindfoot alignment abnormalities, portends a poor prognosis with a high rate of progression to osteoarthritis.[73]

Conservative management is appropriate for smaller, stable OLTs.[74] However, a high number of these lesions may fail nonsurgical management and should be evaluated for surgery.[75] Furthermore, in meta-analysis, 45% of all OLTs fail nonoperative treatment.[76] Thus, expert consensus has moved toward recommendation of surgical management of lesions involving a disrupted subchondral plate. Spontaneous healing may be less predictable, given synovial fluid infiltration into the fissure created by the OLT, which is exacerbated with loading cycles during ambulation and activity.[77] The subsequent high intraosseous pressure underlying the lesion can lead to cyst formation, contributing to pain, unsupported cartilage, and further degenerative change.[78] Thus, surgical management for OLT stabilization is thought to result in improved outcomes and delayed onset of osteoarthritis. Multiple investigators have confirmed these presuppositions.

Several patient-specific factors have been found to impact outcomes after treatment for OLT. Increasing age[79–82] and higher BMI[81] have been implicated for portending inferior outcomes after arthroscopic marrow stimulation. Other investigators have reported contradictory results. Choi and colleagues found that increased age was not an independent risk factor for poor clinical outcomes after arthroscopic treatment of OLT. The study found that older patients had smaller lesions, decreased incidence of trauma, increased duration of symptoms, and more associated intra-articular lesions.[83] Moreover, patient-specific anatomic factors such as hindfoot alignment, ankle stability, and concomitant injuries (while outside the scope of this review) must be assessed and addressed to ensure optimal outcomes.

Lesion-specific characteristics have been shown to predict clinical outcomes. Multiple reports have demonstrated a correlation between size of lesion and outcome, with large lesions shown to have inferior results after surgery.[79–81,84,85] Cuttica and colleagues found that lesions larger than 1.5 cm^2 (determined on MRI) and uncontained lesions were the greatest predictor of poor clinical outcomes.[80] This finding may be the result of altered contact area and contact pressures within the joint that occur with large osteochondral lesions.[86] In addition, deeper lesions which penetrate the subchondral bone and lesions, which are medially located may be poor prognostic factors.[82] Uncontained lesions that involve the shoulder of the talar dome and lack a stable border of articular cartilage do not make suitable candidates for BMS procedures due to exposure to greater stresses during weight-bearing, making fibrocartilage formation less likely to form.[79,80] Hunt and colleagues demonstrated that contact stresses occur closer to the rim of an OLT when the defect reached a diameter of 10 mm and greater. The investigators postulated that this finding coupled with reduced tibiotalar contact area and increasing defect size may contribute to formation of progressively larger defects, subchondral cysts, and increased pain.[87]

With regard to outcomes after specific surgical treatments for OLTs, surgery outperforms conservative care for unstable OLTs. However, determining superiority of one procedural treatment option over another has proved difficult. Direct cartilage repair using k-wire or other fixation techniques, BMS, AMIC, autologous chondrocyte implantation (ACI), application of various biologic adjuncts, and autograft, and allograft options have all demonstrated success in treatment of OLTs.[64,88–108] Van Bergen and colleagues reported good or excellent long-term clinical outcomes in 74% to 78% of patients treated with arthroscopic debridement and BMS with 67% of the patients having no radiographic progression of osteoarthritis at 12 year mean follow-up.[109]

Efforts at pooled meta-analysis have attempted to determine superiority of one OLT treatment option over another. Dahmen and colleagues present a systematic review with meta-analysis of 52 studies with 1236 primary talar OCDs, including two randomized controlled trials (RCTs). Despite concerns regarding heterogeneity of methodologies presented in the pooled studies and significant variation in reported success rates, these investigators determined no difference between BMS, osteochondral autograft transfer system, and osteoperiosteal cylinder graft insertion. Finally, in the most recent pooled analysis comparing treatment options for OLTs, Hongbo and colleagues demonstrate superiority of cartilage regeneration including ACI, matrix-induced autologous chondrocyte implantation (MACI), platelet-rich plasma, and bone marrow-derived cell transplantation and cartilage replacement (including OAT) over microfracture and retrograde drilling.[110–112] However, these findings, while encouraging for the use of cartilage regenerative techniques over isolated microfracture, are limited by the inclusion of lower level studies. Further work including high-level studies and RCTs will be required to make a conclusive differentiation between the current existing treatment options for unstable OLTs.

CLINICS CARE POINTS

- Osteochondral lesions of the talus (OLTs) most commonly occur following a traumatic insult, most often ankle sprains.
- Four staging systems have been described that classify OLTs based on different imaging modalities.
- Conservative treatment of OLTs is reserved for asymptomatic lesions and lesions found incidentally; surgical treatment is recommended for acute displaced osteochondral fragments and symptomatic lesions after failed conservative treatment.
- There remains room for improvement regarding treatment algorithms for OLTs.

ACKNOWLEDGMENTS

The authors would like to thank Dr Annunziato Ned Amendola for his expertise and assistance throughout all aspects of our study and for their help in writing the manuscript.

DISCLOSURE

All authors have no relevant disclosures.

REFERENCES

1. Rosen M. Occult osseous lesions documented by MRI associated with anterior cruciate ligament ruptures. Arthroscopy 1991;7:745–51.
2. Yao L, Lee J. Occult intraosseous fracture: detection with MR imaging. Radiology 1988;167(3):749–51.
3. Powers RT, Dowd TC, Giza E. Surgical treatment for osteochondral lesions of the talus. Arthrosc J Arthrosc Relat Surg 2021;37(12):3393–6.
4. Wang C-C, Yang K-C, Chen H. Current treatment concepts for osteochondral lesions of the talus. Tzu Chi Med J 2021;33(3):243.
5. Dahmen J, Lambers KT, Reilingh ML, et al. No superior treatment for primary osteochondral defects of the talus. Knee Surg Sports Traumatol Arthrosc 2018;26: 2142–57.
6. Thomas M, Jordan M, Hamborg-Petersen E. Arthroscopic treatment of chondral lesions of the ankle joint. evidence based therapy. Unfallchirurg 2016;119(2): 100–8.
7. Ozcan S, Kockara N, Camurcu Y, et al. Magnetic resonance imaging and outcomes of osteochondral lesions of the talus associated with ankle fractures. Foot Ankle Int 2020;41(19):1219–25.

8. Hintermann B, Regazzoni P, Lampert C, et al. Arthroscopic findings in acute fractures of the ankle. Bone Joint Surg Br 2000;82(3):345–51.

9. Aktas S, Kocaoglu B, Gereli A, et al. Incidence of chondral lesions of talar dome in ankle fracture types. Foot Ankle Int 2008;29(3):287–92.

10. Waterman B, Owens B, Davey S, et al. The epidemiology of ankle sprains in the United States. J Bone Joint Surg Am 2010;92(13):2279–84.

11. Doherty C, Delahunt E, Caulfield B, et al. The incidence and prevalence of ankle sprain injury: a systematic review and meta-analysis of prospective epidemiological studies. Sports Med 2014;44(1):123–40.

12. McCollum G, Calder J, Longo U, et al. Talus osteochondral bruises and defects: diagnosis and differentiation. Foot Ankle Clin 2013;18(1):35–47.

13. O'Loughlin P, Heyworth B, Kennedy J. Current concepts in the diagnosis and treatment of osteochondral lesions of the ankle. Am J Sports Med 2010;38(2): 392–404.

14. Berndt AL, Harty M. Transchondral fractures (osteochondritis dissecans) of the talus. J Bone Joint Surg Am 1959;41-A:988–1020.

15. van Dijk CN, Reilingh ML, Zengerink M, et al. Osteochondral defects in the ankle: why painful? Knee Surg Sports Traumatol Arthrosc 2010;18(5):570–80.

16. Ferkel RD, Zanotti RM, Komenda GA, et al. Arthroscopic treatment of chronic osteochondral lesions of the talus: long-term results. Am J Sports Med 2008; 36(9):1750–62.

17. Looze C, Capo J, Ryan M, et al. Evaluation and Management of Osteochondral Lesions of the Talus. Cartilage 2017;8(1):19–30.

18. Pick M. Familial osteochondritis dissecans. J Bone Joint Surg Br 1955;37(1B): 142–5.

19. Mubarak S, Carroll N. Familial osteochondritis dissecans of the knee. Clin Orthop Relat Res 1979;140:131–6.

20. Gerber J, Williams G, Scoville C, et al. Persistent disability associated with ankle sprains: a prospective examination of an athletic population. Foot Ankle Int 1998;19:653–60.

21. van Rijn R, van Os A, Bernsen R, et al. What is the clinical course of acute ankle sprains? A systematic literature review. Am J Med 2008;121:324–31.

22. Takao M, Uchio Y, Naito K, et al. Arthroscopic assessment for intra-articular disorders in residual ankle disability after sprain. Am J Sports Med 2005;33(5): 686–92.

23. Taga I, Shino K, Inoue M, et al. Articular cartilage lesions in ankles with lateral ligament injury. An arthroscopic study. Am J Sports Med 1993;21(1):120–6.

24. van Dijk C, Bossuyt P, Marti R. Medial ankle pain after lateral ligament rupture. J Bone Joint Surg Br 1996;78:562–7.

25. Miklovic T, Donovan L, Protzuk O, et al. Acute lateral ankle sprain to chronic ankle instability: a pathway of dysfunction. Phys Sportsmed 2017;46(1):116–22.

26. Odak S, Ahluwalia R, Shivarathre D, et al. Arthroscopic evaluation of impingement and osteochondral lesions in chronic lateral ankle instability. Foot Ankle Int 2015;36(9):1045–9.

27. Hepple S, Winson IG, Glew D. Osteochondral lesions of the talus: a revised classification. Foot Ankle Int 1999;20(12):789–93.

28. Verhagen RA, Maas M, Dijkgraaf MG, et al. Prospective study on diagnostic strategies in osteochondral lesions of the talus. Is MRI superior to helical CT? J Bone Joint Surg Br 2005;87(1):41–6.

29. Flick AB, Gould N. Osteochondritis dissecans of the talus (transchondral fractures of the talus): review of the literature and new surgical approach for medial dome lesions. Foot Ankle 1985;5(4):165–85.

30. Loomer R, Fisher C, Lloyd-Smith R, et al. Osteochondral lesions of the talus. Am J Sports Med 1993;21(1):13–9.

31. Thompson JP, Loomer RL. Osteochondral lesions of the talus in a sports medicine clinic. A new radiographic technique and surgical approach. Am J Sports Med 1984;12(6):460–3.

32. van Bergen CJ, Gerards RM, Opdam KT, et al. Diagnosing, planning and evaluating osteochondral ankle defects with imaging modalities. World J Orthop 2015;6(11):944–53.

33. van Bergen CJ, Tuijthof GJ, Blankevoort L, et al. Computed tomography of the ankle in full plantar flexion: a reliable method for preoperative planning of arthroscopic access to osteochondral defects of the talus. Arthroscopy 2012;28(7):985–92.

34. Nakasa T, Ikuta Y, Yoshikawa M, et al. Added value of preoperative computed tomography for determining cartilage degeneration in patients with osteochondral lesions of the talar dome. Am J Sports Med 2018;46(1):208–16.

35. Nakasa T, Adachi N, Kato T, et al. Appearance of subchondral bone in computed tomography is related to cartilage damage in osteochondral lesions of the talar dome. Foot Ankle Int 2014;35(6):600–6.

36. Uozumi H, Sugita T, Aizawa T, et al. Histologic findings and possible causes of osteochondritis dissecans of the knee. Am J Sports Med 2009;37(10):2003–8.

37. Tazegul TE, Anderson DD, Barbachan Mansur NS, et al. An objective computational method to quantify ankle osteoarthritis from low-dose weightbearing computed tomography. Foot Ankle Orthop 2022;7(3). https://doi.org/10.1177/24730114221116805. 24730114221116805.

38. Lintz F, Ricard C, Mehdi N, et al. Hindfoot alignment assessment by the foot-ankle offset: a diagnostic study. Arch Orthop Trauma Surg 2023;143(5):2373–82.

39. Day MA, Ho M, Dibbern K, et al. Correlation of 3D Joint space width from weightbearing CT with outcomes after intra-articular calcaneal fracture. Foot Ankle Int 2020;41(9):1106–16.

40. De Smet AA, Fisher DR, Burnstein MI, et al. Value of MR imaging in staging osteochondral lesions of the talus (osteochondritis dissecans): results in 14 patients. AJR Am J Roentgenol 1990;154(3):555–8.

41. Magee TH, Hinson GW. Usefulness of MR imaging in the detection of talar dome injuries. AJR Am J Roentgenol 1998;170(5):1227–30.

42. Loredo R, Sanders TG. Imaging of osteochondral injuries. Clin Sports Med 2001;20(2):249–78.

43. Raikin SM, Elias I, Zoga AC, et al. Osteochondral lesions of the talus: localization and morphologic data from 424 patients using a novel anatomical grid scheme. Foot Ankle Int 2007;28(2):154–61.

44. Mintz DN, Tashjian GS, Connell DA, et al. Osteochondral lesions of the talus: a new magnetic resonance grading system with arthroscopic correlation. Arthroscopy 2003;19(4):353–9.

45. Lee KB, Bai LB, Park JG, et al. A comparison of arthroscopic and MRI findings in staging of osteochondral lesions of the talus. Knee Surg Sports Traumatol Arthrosc 2008;16(11):1047–51.

46. Tan TC, Wilcox DM, Frank L, et al. MR imaging of articular cartilage in the ankle: comparison of available imaging sequences and methods of measurement in cadavers. Skeletal Radiol 1996;25(8):749–55.
47. Leumann A, Valderrabano V, Plaass C, et al. A novel imaging method for osteochondral lesions of the talus–comparison of SPECT-CT with MRI. Am J Sports Med 2011;39(5):1095–101.
48. D'Ambrosi R, Maccario C, Ursino C, et al. The role of bone marrow edema on osteochondral lesions of the talus. Foot Ankle Surg 2018;24(3):229–35.
49. Pritsch M, Horoshovski H, Farine I. Arthroscopic treatment of osteochondral lesions of the talus. JBJS 1986;68(6):862–5.
50. Dombrowski ME, Yasui Y, Murawski CD, et al. Conservative management and biological treatment strategies: proceedings of the international consensus meeting on cartilage repair of the ankle. Foot Ankle Int 2018;39(1_suppl): 9S–15S.
51. Amendola A, Lee KB, Saltzman CL, et al. Technique and early experience with posterior arthroscopic subtalar arthrodesis. Foot Ankle Int 2007;28(3):298–302.
52. Willits K, Sonneveld H, Amendola A, et al. Outcome of posterior ankle arthroscopy for hindfoot impingement. Arthrosc J Arthrosc Relat Surg 2008;24(2): 196–202.
53. Muir D, Saltzman CL, Tochigi Y, et al. Talar dome access for osteochondral lesions. Am J Sports Med 2006;34(9):1457–63.
54. Alexander IJ, Watson JT. Step-cut osteotomy of the medial malleolus for exposure of the medial ankle joint space. Foot Ankle 1991;11(4):242–3.
55. Draper SD, Fallat LM. Autogenous bone grafting for the treatment of talar dome lesions. J Foot Ankle Surg 2000;39(1):15–23.
56. Kumai T, Takakura Y, Higashiyama I, et al. Arthroscopic drilling for the treatment of osteochondral lesions of the talus. J Bone Joint Surg Am 1999;81(9):1229–35.
57. Tochigi Y, Amendola A, Muir D, et al. Surgical approach for centrolateral talar osteochondral lesions with an anterolateral osteotomy. Foot Ankle Int 2002; 23(11):1038–9.
58. Anders S, Lechler P, Rackl W, et al. Fluoroscopy-guided retrograde core drilling and cancellous bone grafting in osteochondral defects of the talus. Int Orthop 2012;36(8):1635–40.
59. Geerling J, Zech S, Kendoff D, et al. Initial outcomes of 3-dimensional imaging-based computer-assisted retrograde drilling of talar osteochondral lesions. Am J Sports Med 2009;37(7):1351–7.
60. Kono M, Takao M, Naito K, et al. Retrograde drilling for osteochondral lesions of the talar dome. Am J Sports Med 2006;34(9):1450–6.
61. Smyth NA, Zwiers R, Wiegerinck JI, et al. Posterior hindfoot arthroscopy: A review. Review. Am J Sports Med 2014;42(1):225–34.
62. Reilingh ML, Van Sterkenburg MN, De Leeuw PAJ, et al. Ankle arthroscopy: Indications, techniques and complications. Article. SA Orthop J 2009;2(8):51–8.
63. Van Dijk CN, Van Bergen CJA. Advancements in ankle arthroscopy. review. J Am Acad Orthop Surg 2008;16(11):635–46.
64. Dekker TJ, Dekker PK, Tainter DM, et al. Treatment of osteochondral lesions of the talus: a critical analysis review. JBJS Rev 2017;5(3). https://doi.org/10.2106/JBJS.RVW.16.00065.
65. Al-Shaikh RA, Chou LB, Mann JA, et al. Autologous osteochondral grafting for talar cartilage defects. Foot Ankle Int 2002;23(5):381–9.
66. Baltzer AW, Arnold JP. Bone-cartilage transplantation from the ipsilateral knee for chondral lesions of the talus. Arthroscopy 2005;21(2):159–66.

67. Hangody L, Kish G, Módis L, et al. Mosaicplasty for the treatment of osteochondritis dissecans of the talus: two to seven year results in 36 patients. Foot Ankle Int 2001;22(7):552–8.

68. Gautier E, Kolker D, Jakob RP. Treatment of cartilage defects of the talus by autologous osteochondral grafts. J Bone Joint Surg Br 2002;84(2):237–44.

69. Raikin SM. Fresh osteochondral allografts for large-volume cystic osteochondral defects of the talus. J Bone Joint Surg Am 2009;91(12):2818–26.

70. Williams SK, Amiel D, Ball ST, et al. Prolonged storage effects on the articular cartilage of fresh human osteochondral allografts. J Bone Joint Surg Am 2003;85(11):2111–20.

71. Sijbrandij ES, van Gils APG, Louwerens JWK, et al. Posttraumatic Subchondral Bone Contusions and Fractures of the Talotibial Joint. Am J Roentgenol 2000; 175(6):1707–10.

72. Seo SG, Kim JS, Seo DK, et al. Osteochondral lesions of the talus. Acta Orthop 2018;89(4):462–7.

73. Krause F, Anwander H. Osteochondral lesion of the talus: still a problem? EFORT Open Rev 2022;7(6):337–43.

74. Badekas T, Takvorian M, Souras N. Treatment principles for osteochondral lesions in foot and ankle. Int Orthop 2013;37(9):1697–706.

75. Schachter AK, Chen AL, Reddy PD, et al. Osteochondral lesions of the talus. J Am Acad Orthop Surg May-Jun 2005;13(3):152–8.

76. Tol JL, Struijs PA, Bossuyt PM, et al. Treatment strategies in osteochondral defects of the talar dome: a systematic review. Foot Ankle Int 2000;21(2):119–26.

77. Nakamae A, Engebretsen L, Bahr R, et al. Natural history of bone bruises after acute knee injury: clinical outcome and histopathological findings. Knee Surg Sports Traumatol Arthrosc 2006;14(12):1252–8.

78. Shapiro F, Koide S, Glimcher MJ. Cell origin and differentiation in the repair of full-thickness defects of articular cartilage. JBJS 1993;75(4).

79. Deol PP, Cuttica DJ, Smith WB, et al. Osteochondral lesions of the talus: size, age, and predictors of outcomes. Foot Ankle Clin 2013;18(1):13–34.

80. Cuttica DJ, Smith WB, Hyer CF, et al. Osteochondral lesions of the talus: predictors of clinical outcome. Foot Ankle Int 2011;32(11):1045–51.

81. Chuckpaiwong B, Berkson EM, Theodore GH. Microfracture for osteochondral lesions of the ankle: outcome analysis and outcome predictors of 105 cases. Arthroscopy 2008;24(1):106–12.

82. Yoshimura I, Kanazawa K, Takeyama A, et al. Arthroscopic bone marrow stimulation techniques for osteochondral lesions of the talus: prognostic factors for small lesions. Am J Sports Med 2013;41(3):528–34.

83. Choi WJ, Kim BS, Lee JW. Osteochondral lesion of the talus: could age be an indication for arthroscopic treatment? Am J Sports Med 2012;40(2):419–24.

84. Gobbi A, Francisco RA, Lubowitz JH, et al. Osteochondral lesions of the talus: randomized controlled trial comparing chondroplasty, microfracture, and osteochondral autograft transplantation. Arthroscopy 2006;22:1085–92.

85. Choi WJ, Park KK, Kim BS, et al. Osteochondral lesion of the talus:is there a critical defect size for poor outcome? Am J Sports Med 2009;37(10):1974–80.

86. Christensen J, Driscoll H, Tencer A. 1994 William J. Stickel Gold Award. Contact characteristics of the ankle joint. Part 2. The effects of talar dome cartilage defects. J Am Podiatr Med Assoc 1994;84(11):537–47.

87. Hunt KJ, Lee AT, Lindsey DP, et al. Osteochondral lesions of the talus:effect of defect size and plantarflexion angle on ankle joint stresses. Am J Sports Med 2012;40(4):895–901.

88. Ackermann J, Casari FA, Germann C, et al. Autologous matrix-induced chondrogenesis with lateral ligament stabilization for osteochondral lesions of the talus in patients with ankle instability. Orthop J Sports Med 2021;9(5). https://doi.org/10.1177/23259671211007439. 23259671211007439.

89. Adams SB Jr, Demetracopoulos CA, Parekh SG, et al. Arthroscopic particulated juvenile cartilage allograft transplantation for the treatment of osteochondral lesions of the talus. Arthrosc Tech 2014;3(4):e533–7.

90. Ahmad J, Maltenfort M. Arthroscopic treatment of osteochondral lesions of the talus with allograft cartilage matrix. Foot Ankle Int 2017;38(8):855–62.

91. Ahn J, Choi JG, Jeong BO. Clinical outcomes after arthroscopic microfracture for osteochondral lesions of the talus are better in patients with decreased postoperative subchondral bone marrow edema. Knee Surg Sports Traumatol Arthrosc 2021;29(5):1570–6.

92. Arshad Z, Aslam A, Iqbal AM, et al. Should arthroscopic bone marrow stimulation be used in the management of secondary osteochondral lesions of the talus? a systematic review. Clin Orthop Relat Res 2022;480(6):1112–25.

93. Ayyaswamy B, Salim M, Sidaginamale R, et al. Early to medium term outcomes of osteochondral lesions of the talus treated by autologous matrix induced chondrogenesis (AMIC). Foot Ankle Surg 2021;27(2):207–12.

94. Casari FA, Germann C, Weigelt L, et al. The role of magnetic resonance imaging in autologous matrix-induced chondrogenesis for osteochondral lesions of the talus: analyzing MOCART 1 and 2.0. Cartilage 2021;13(1_suppl):639S–45S.

95. Cerrato R. Particulated juvenile articular cartilage allograft transplantation for osteochondral lesions of the talus. Foot Ankle Clin 2013;18(1):79–87.

96. Chen W, Tang K, Yuan C, et al. Intermediate results of large cystic medial osteochondral lesions of the talus treated with osteoperiosteal cylinder autografts from the medial tibia. Arthroscopy 2015;31(8):1557–64.

97. Choi JI, Lee KB. Comparison of clinical outcomes between arthroscopic subchondral drilling and microfracture for osteochondral lesions of the talus. Knee Surg Sports Traumatol Arthrosc 2016;24(7):2140–7.

98. Corr D, Raikin J, O'Neil J, et al. Long-term outcomes of microfracture for treatment of osteochondral lesions of the talus. Foot Ankle Int 2021;42(7):833–40.

99. Correa Bellido P, Wadhwani J, Gil Monzo E. Matrix-induced autologous chondrocyte implantation grafting in osteochondral lesions of the talus: evaluation of cartilage repair using T2 mapping. J Orthop 2019;16(6):500–3.

100. de l'Escalopier N, Amouyel T, Mainard D, et al. Long-term outcome for repair of osteochondral lesions of the talus by osteochondral autograft: a series of 56 Mosaicplasties(R). Orthop Traumatol Surg Res 2021;107(8S):103075.

101. Deng E, Shi W, Jiang Y, et al. Comparison of autologous osteoperiosteal cylinder and osteochondral graft transplantation in the treatment of large cystic osteochondral lesions of the talus (OLTs): a protocol for a non-inferiority randomised controlled trial. BMJ Open 2020;10(2):e033850.

102. Dilley JE, Everhart JS, Klitzman RG. Hyaluronic acid as an adjunct to microfracture in the treatment of osteochondral lesions of the talus: a systematic review of randomized controlled trials. BMC Musculoskelet Disord 2022;23(1):313.

103. Ettinger S, Stukenborg-Colsman C, Waizy H, et al. Results of HemiCAP((R)) implantation as a salvage procedure for osteochondral lesions of the talus. J Foot Ankle Surg Jul-Aug 2017;56(4):788–92.

104. Flynn S, Ross KA, Hannon CP, et al. Autologous Osteochondral Transplantation for Osteochondral Lesions of the Talus. Foot Ankle Int 2016;37(4):363–72.

105. Fu S, Yang K, Li X, et al. Radiographic and clinical outcomes after arthroscopic microfracture for osteochondral lesions of the talus: 5-year results in 355 consecutive ankles. Orthop J Sports Med 2022;10(10). https://doi.org/10.1177/23259671221128772. 23259671221128772.
106. Gao F, Chen N, Sun W, et al. Combined therapy with shock wave and retrograde bone marrow-derived cell transplantation for osteochondral lesions of the talus. Sci Rep 2017;7(1):2106.
107. Gaul F, Tirico LEP, McCauley JC, et al. Osteochondral allograft transplantation for osteochondral lesions of the talus: midterm follow-up. Foot Ankle Int 2019; 40(2):202–9.
108. Georgiannos D, Bisbinas I, Badekas A. Osteochondral transplantation of autologous graft for the treatment of osteochondral lesions of talus: 5- to 7-year follow-up. Knee Surg Sports Traumatol Arthrosc 2016;24(12):3722–9.
109. van Bergen CJ, Kox LS, Maas M, et al. Arthroscopic treatment of osteochondral defects of the talus: outcomes at eight to twenty years of follow-up. JBJS 2013; 95(6):519–25.
110. Tan H, Li A, Qiu X, et al. Operative treatments for osteochondral lesions of the talus in adults: A systematic review and meta-analysis. Medicine 2021; 100(25):e26330.
111. Delco ML, Kennedy JG, Bonassar LJ, et al. Post-traumatic osteoarthritis of the ankle: A distinct clinical entity requiring new research approaches. J Orthop Res 2017;35(3):440–53.
112. Pathria MN, Chung CB, Resnick DL. Acute and stress-related injuries of bone and cartilage: pertinent anatomy, basic biomechanics, and imaging perspective. Radiology 2016;280(1):21–38.

Osteochondral Lesion of the Talus

Quality of Life, Lesion Site, and Lesion Size

Tania Szejnfeld Mann, MD, PhD[a,1], Caio Nery, MD, PhD[b,*]

KEYWORDS

- Osteochondral lesions • Osteochondritis dissecans • Talus • Foot and ankle
- Cartilage damage • Subchondral bone • OLT size • OLT site

KEY POINTS

- Osteochondral lesion of the talus (OLT) is one of the most common causes of persistent pain at the ankle joint after an ankle sprain and is associated with the degradation of quality of life.
- Two-thirds of the lesions (73%) are located on the medial part of the talus, 28% of the lesions are posteromedial and 31% centromedial.
- Size is one of the most relevant predictors of poor outcome; OLT of up to 100 mm^2 can behave in a more indolent condition.

INTRODUCTION

Osteochondral lesions of the talus (OLTs) are, by definition, lesions that affect the articular cartilage and the subchondral bone of the talus.[1] The term subchondral bone encompasses both the subchondral plate and the medullary region of the talus, where the presence of different degrees of edema or cyst formation provides us with important information about the intensity and chronicity of the regional pathologic process and, consequently, about the prognosis of the lesion[1] and its potential influence on patient outcomes and quality of life. Most common associations are ankle instability and previous ankle trauma, reported at almost 80% of the cases.[2]

First described in the knee, by König, in 1888,[3] as osteochondritis dissecans, and later described by Kappis in the talar dome,[4] the exact cause of these lesions still remains controversial.

[a] Orthopedic Surgery, Federal University of São Paulo, Escola Paulista de Medicina, Sao Paulo, Brazil; [b] Orthopedics and Traumatology, UNIFESP, Federal University of São Paulo, Brazil
[1] Present address: Avenida Agami, 80 apt 71. Moema. São Paulo/SP. ZIP 04522-000, Brazil.
* Corresponding author. AV. Albert Einstein, 627 - Bl. A1 -#317, Morumbi, São Paulo/SP 05652-000, Brazil
E-mail address: caionerymd@gmail.com

Foot Ankle Clin N Am 29 (2024) 213–224
https://doi.org/10.1016/j.fcl.2023.07.007
1083-7515/24/© 2023 Elsevier Inc. All rights reserved.

Within the recent years, the first hypothesis of a vascular infraction as the main cause of the OLT has been replaced by the Van Dijk's hypothesis that points to shearing forces as responsible for the cartilage damage and to the bone contusion resulting from a high-impact force as the forerunner of a subchondral defect.[5,6]

Traumatic cartilage injuries can comprise 3 categories: microdamage or blunt trauma, chondral fractures, and osteochondral fractures.[7] When there is dissipation of forces throughout the cartilage, subchondral plate can be damaged. Traumatic insult has been related to 93% to 98% of lateral defects and 61% to 70% of medial defects.[8]

When ankle is repeatedly loaded, the articular fluids are squeezed out of the cartilage into the subchondral bone promoting pain and progressive increase in flow of this liquid to the subchondral plate. There is an inverse proportion of pressure and size of the defect. The smaller the opening at the subchondral bone, the higher is the pressure at the subchondral region.

According to van Dijk's observations, the pain that characterizes OLT has its genesis in the increase in hydrostatic pressure in the medullary region of the talus, determined by the fluid hyper flow in the area and which stimulates the numerous sensory nerve endings existing there (**Fig. 1**).[5]

Quality of Life

Ankle sprain is one the most frequent musculoskeletal injury in lower limbs. Worldwide, approximately 712,000 individuals sprain their ankles each day.[9] Most of the sprains are assisted by a general orthopedic doctor and often dismissed as trivial injuries, thought to resolve quickly with minimal treatment. However, feelings of instability and recurrent ankle sprain injuries (termed chronic ankle instability, or CAI) have been reported in up to 70% of patients.[10] CAI by itself, even without the accompanying complications, already constitutes an important factor in reducing quality of life. OLT may occur in up to 50% of acute ankle sprains and fractures, particularly in association with sports injuries[11] and represents one of the main causes of persistent pain.

OLT is a predominantly male disease that affects individuals in their thirties.[12,13] In general, symptoms develop between 6 and 12 months after the index trauma (ankle sprain or fracture) and are characterized by locoregional pain, tenderness, and deep swelling on the lateral or medial sides of the ankle. These symptoms are directly related to high-impact physical activities and body weight support.[14]

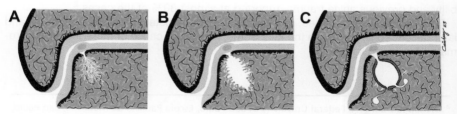

Fig. 1. Van Dijk's theory to explain the genesis of pain in osteochondral lesions of the talus. (A) When cartilage impermeability is compromised by a trauma that corrupts the SBP, synovial fluid flows into the bone marrow. In the beginning, the infiltration is smooth and reticular; (B) With the constant load of the body weight, the flow and pressure of the fluids pumped to the medullary region increases; (C) As the condition progresses, multiple medullary cysts are formed with sclerosis of their borders and channels that communicate with accessory chambers. Pain is generated by this process, which ends up reaching the numerous nerve endings in the bone marrow of the talus.

Interestingly, most of these patients have only mild ankle synovitis, which is not related to the genesis of joint pain, which depends almost exclusively on activity and load on the lesion site. Chronic lesions classically present as deep lateral or medial ankle pain worsened by weight-bearing. Mild swelling, ankle stiffness, and diminished range of motion can be present (**Fig. 2**). For all these reasons, as a rule, the clinical examination does not provide reliable information about the characteristics of the osteochondral lesion, and the absence of these symptoms does not rule out an osteochondral defect.[15]

OLT are associated with degradation of quality of life. In a retrospective study that included 52 patients with symptomatic OLT for more than 6 months, Usuelli and colleagues assessed OLT and quality of life using SF-12, divided into physical component summary (PCS) and mental component summary (MCS).[16] Authors observed that mean MCS and PCS resulted in 43.9 and 32.5, respectively. When comparing these results with similar general population with no pathology, patients had a mean MCS of 50.8 and PCS of 52.9.[17] And patients with lombosciatalgia presented MCS of 45.7 and PCS of 43.1. These results show that OLTs affect the quality of life similarly to the disability associated with other orthopedics such as lombosciatalgia.[16]

Nonoperative treatment can present improvement in pain and quality of life in patients presenting small defects. Seo and colleagues followed 244 patients for a mean time of 6 years (3–10).[18] From 244 patients diagnosed with OLT, 217 (89%)

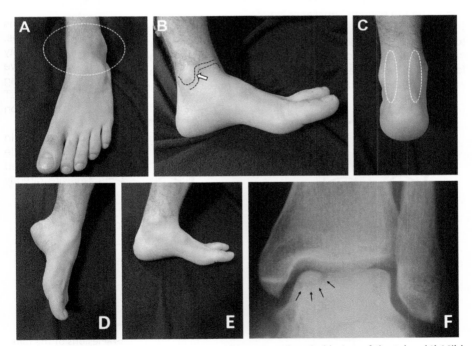

Fig. 2. Clinical aspect of a young patient with an osteochondral lesion of the talus: (*A*) Mild and nonspecific swelling of the anterior region of the ankle; (*B*) Painful area of the medial "soft spot" of the ankle where the positive Drennan sign is observed in the medial OLT (*white arrow*); (*C*) Slight blurring of the lateral and medial posterior gutters due to the slight peri-articular edema; (*D*) Good mobility in plantar flexion; (*E*) Slight limitation of dorsiflexion; and (*F*) Plain radiography (AP) of the left ankle of the same patient, where the presence of a medial OLT can be clearly observed (*black arrows*).

received nonoperative treatment. Treatment consisted of unlimited daily activity and use of non-steroidal anti-inflammatory drugs (NSAIDs) as needed for intermittent pain. Initially, the mean width, length, and depth measurements of OLT were 6.9 (1.7–13.1) mm, 9.4 (1.9–19.2) mm, and 5.4 (1.0–15.5) mm, respectively. Most of the patients had no change in lesion size, and weight-bearing radiographs did not demonstrate progression of ankle osteoarthritis. The mean VAS score decreased from 3.8 (1–8) at the initial visit to 0.9 (0–4) at the final follow-up (P < .001). The mean American Orthopedic Foot and Ankle Society (AOFAS) ankle–hindfoot score improved from 86 (41–93) at the initial visit to 93 (65–100) at the final follow-up (P <.001). The mean SF-36 score increased from 52 (30–90) to 71 (37–97) (P < .001). Only 9 patients reported limitation of their preferred sports activity. In female patients, SF-36 scores were lower at final follow-up than in male patients (P = .01); however, there was no significant correlation between AOFAS ankle–hindfoot scores and sex (P = .2) or age (P = .05).

Lesion Site

Historically, talar lesions were described as located in the posteromedial or anterolateral portions of the talar dome, with the posteromedial lesions being deeper and cup-shaped in morphology, and with anterolateral lesions typically shallower and wafer-shaped. Accompanying this description, became current the notion that posteromedial lesions were more difficult to treat, evolving with worse outcomes and greater impact on the patients' quality of life.[19]

In 2007, Raikin and colleagues established a 9-zone grid system on the talar dome to accurately describe the exact location of these lesions and typical morphologic characteristics for each common location on the talar dome surface.[20] Articular surface of the talar dome was divided in 3 columns and 3 rows in axial plane. Nine equal zones were assigned and numbered from 1 to 9, starting medial and anterior (**Fig. 3**).

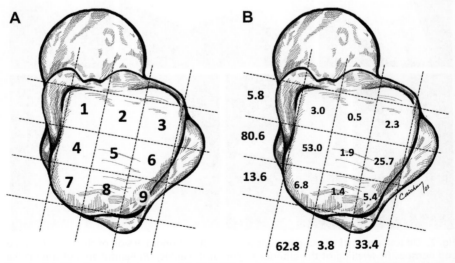

Figs. 3. (A) The 9-zone anatomic grid of Raikin and colleagues recommended for locating osteochondral lesions of the talus. Numbering begins with the anteromedial area and ends with the posterolateral area of the talus; (B) Frequency of lesions according to Raikin's areas, observed in 428 lesions of 424 patients. Lesions occur more frequently in the medial (areas 1, 4 and 7 - 62.8%) and (areas 4, 5 and 6 - 80.6%) and in the equatorial areas (4%, 5%, and 6%–80.6%) of the talus.

Authors identified 63% of lesions on medial talar dome (zones 1, 4, and 7), and 33% involving lateral talar dome (zones 3, 6, and 9). Only 3.7% of the lesions were located at the central column (zones 2, 5, and 8). Regarding anteroposterior plane, 80% were located at the central third (zones 4, 5, and 6). Medial central talar dome (zone 4) was most frequently involved (53.0%), followed by lateral central (zone 6) in 25% of the cases. Same study stated that medial talar dome lesions also presented different characteristics from the lateral talar dome ones. Medial lesions presented larger in surface area and deeper than lateral defects. In medial talar dome, osteochondral lesion mean area was 93.1 mm^2, compared with a mean surface area of 60.1 mm^2 for lateral lesions ($P < .01$).

This grid system allowed to identify that OCL are more central, with greatest incidence concentrated at zones 4 and 7, rather than at zones 3 and 7, as described by Berndt and Harty.

A recent metanalysis included 51 articles and reported a total of 2087 lesions in 2066 ankles of 2054 patients.[2] Studies included classified OLT according to the grid system described by Raikin. The average age of the studied patients was 37 (range, 13–55) years. There was a similar gender distribution with 1212 (59%) male patients and 842 (41%) female patients. The average preoperative lesion size was 86 mm^2 (range, 44–250). Most frequently examination used to investigate lesions were a combination of either x-ray and MRI or MRI and computed tomography (CT), in 43% of the cases. Two-thirds of the lesions were located on the medial part of the talus (73%). Twenty-eight percent of the lesions were in the posteromedial (zone 7) and 31% centromedial (zone 4). Together, all lateral lesions summed 24%, and central lesions 5% of all lesions described (see **Fig. 3**). Medial OLT sized up to 104 mm^2 (92–104 mm^2, whereas lateral lesions tended to be wider (92–154 mm^2), and central ones even wider (134–205 mm^2).

Kim and colleagues,[21] interested in the correlation between lateral CAI and the OLT characteristics, found that there is a higher prevalence of medial talar lesions (87.9%) than lateral talar lesions (12.1%), and that the cartilage-only lesions are much more frequent than the osteochondral type, 65.4% and 34.8%, respectively. The mean lesion size was significantly larger in female patients (113.9 + 28.4 mm^2) than in male patients (100.7 + 18.0 mm^2). The mean lesion size was also significantly larger in patients who enjoyed a high level of sports activity or engaged in heavy work level. This study highlights that women engaged in high level of sports or heavy work would be more likely to develop medial OLT following a traumatic injury of the ankle.

Lesion Size

Weight-bearing radiographs are indicated as a primary imaging modality. Ankle antero-posterior and lateral views and ankle mortise views are routinely used but plain radiographs are insensitive and provide only unidimensional measures of OLT[22] and almost 50% of ankle osteochondral lesions can be missed.[13]

In 1959, Berndt and Harty described a simple 4-part classification for OLT, based on radiographic findings, that they believed represented increasing severity of the lesion.[19] Berndt and Harty's classification consider stages 1 to 4. Stage 1 represents trabecular compression of subchondral bone, Stage 2 a partially detached osteochondral fragment, Stage 3 a completely detached but undisplaced lesion, and Stage 4 a detached and displaced lesion (**Fig. 4**). This classification has been used for several years but more modern imaging techniques such as CT-based imaging (computed tomography [CT], artho-CT, single-photon emission computed tomography [SPECT]-CT) and/or MRI has proved to be better for site and size evaluation.[23] Ankle radiographic images can fail to detect up to 30% to 46% of OLT.[24]

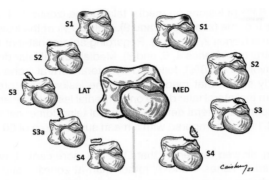

Fig. 4. Description by Berndt and Harty to explain the etiologic mechanism and stages of osteochondral lesions of the talus. On the left-hand side of the figure (LAT), we see the stages of lateral injuries, generally shallower: Stage 1 (S1)—compression of the edge of the talus against the fibula; Stage 2 (S2)—the progression of force causes the avulsion of an osteochondral chip that remains partially connected to the body of the talus; Stage 3 (S3)—the fragment is completely disconnected from the talus but still remains in its original location either (Stage 3a–S3a) or is completely deviated; Stage 4 (S4)–due to total detachment, the osteochondral fragment may be inverted in the lesion bed itself. On the right-hand side of the figure (MED), stages of medial lesions of the talus are shown, which are usually deeper, and dome-shaped. Stage 1 (S1)–The impact of the medial edge of the talus against the tibia produces an area of local compression; The progression of force can generate partial (Stage 2–S2) or total (Stage 3–S3) tearing of an osteochondral chip that remains in its original location; In Stage 4 (S4), the osteochondral fragment no longer maintains any relationship with the site from which it was torn out.

MRI has been accepted as the standard imaging tool with excellent sensitivity and specificity in evaluating cartilage, soft tissue, and subchondral bone, such as subchondral bone marrow edema and cysts, without exposure to radiation.[1,21,25,26] Mintz and colleagues found that MRI allowed correct identification and grading for 33 of 40 (83%) osteochondral lesions, using MRI as imaging tool and arthroscopy as standard.[25]

After 50 years of Berndt and Harty's classification, Hepple and colleagues introduced a specific MRI classification, based on some of the aspects as Berndt and Harty.[19,24] This revised classification uses the same premises and adds author's impression that osteochondral lesions represent a broad spectrum of pathologic condition whereby a lesion can begin at any stage depending on the magnitude of the initial insult and carries the risk of increasing severity. This MRI classification is currently widely used[27] (**Table 1**) (**Fig. 5**).

Table 1	
Hepple's MRI revised grading system[24]	
Stage	**MRI Aspect**
Stage 1	Articular cartilage damage only
Stage 2a	Cartilage injury with underlying fracture and surrounding bone edema
Stage 2b	Without surrounding bone edema
Stage 3	Detached but undispatched fragment
Stage 4	Detached and displaced fragment
Stage 5	Subchondral cyst formation

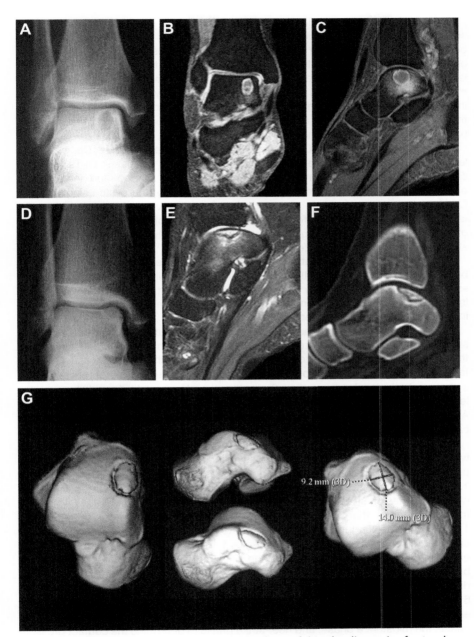

Fig. 5. Imaging diagnosis: (*A*) Plain radiology can be useful in the diagnosis of osteochondral lesions of the talus but its specificity and accuracy are not ideal. In this case, we see the sclerosis that has formed at the periphery of a subchondral cyst in the medial half of the thallus (*B* and *C*). T2-weighted coronal and sagittal MRI sections of the same patient, where the cyst and the extensive medullary edema are clearly seen, which determine intense and constant pain (*D–G*). Plain radiograph (AP), MRI image (sagittal T2 slice), and CT images (sagittal and 3D reconstruction) of a patient with a medial osteochondral lesion of the talus. It is important to realize that the MRI image oversize the lesion but clearly shows medullary

However, MRI might overdiagnose or overestimate the extent of OLT due to bone edema,[28] and CT can provide more precise information than MRI on subchondral bone, such as the size, the shape, bone sclerosis, absorption, the subchondral bone plate (SBP), and cysts. In the pathogenesis of OLT, the importance of the SBP is well discussed. The SBP plays an important role in cartilage metabolism, which means that a damaged SBP is not able to support the overlying cartilage, which results in the loss of proteoglycans and glycoprotein.[29] Nakasa and colleagues demonstrated that CT is a useful tool for the evaluation of subchondral bone and but difficult to evaluate the cartilage surface condition.[28]

Currently, either or MRI or CT can be chosen to study lesion's size. Deng and colleagues compared reliability and validity of MRI and CT in evaluating OLTs with subchondral cysts in 48 patients through 2 experienced blinded and independent observers, who measured the length, width, and depth of the cysts using MRI and CT.[13] Observers achieved an almost perfect interobserver reliability (0.935 < ICC <0.999), with no statistical difference in measurements of length, width, and depth of the lesions. As for comparing both methods to classify the type of lesion, the kappa statistical revealed almost perfect correlation (k = 0.831).[13]

Regarding to the high–weight ratio, Usuelli and colleagues found a linear correlation between body mass index (BMI) and lesion size (square millimeter) measured by MRI, especially OLT located at the equatorial portion of the talus (Raikin zones 4–6).[16] Increased BMI can increase ankle pressure during movements but very few studies investigated that specific aspect.

The size of the lesion may have an effect on patient outcomes because larger lesions can alter the contact stresses of the ankle joint. There is still a debate about the size threshold of the talar osteochondral lesion, which is directly related to less favorable outcomes. In a retrospective analysis that included 120 ankles with OLT symptomatic lesion for more than 6 months, the strongest MRI predictor was the lesion area.[22] Patients with a defect area larger than 150 mm^2 were scored lower AOFAS than 80 points, and the patients with smaller defect areas showed a significantly superior clinical success rate at 48-month follow-up.

Chuckpaiwong and colleagues found that 15 mm was the critical width beyond which bone marrow stimulation (BMS) was associated with a greater likelihood of failure.[30] Cuttica and colleagues described odds of poor outcome increased by 1.42 ± 0.64 for patients with OLT size greater than 1.5 cm^2 when compared with those with smaller lesion sizes, resulting in an odds ratio 4.14 (95% CI; 1.19, 14.44).[31] Authors also found that uncontained lesions increased risk of poor outcomes by 1.44 ± 0.70, resulting in odds ratio of 4.23 (95% CI; 1.083, 16.518). Larger lesions can alter the contact stresses of the ankle joint. Li and colleagues constructed a finite element model of the ankle to explore the influence of the size of defect areas on the biomechanics and stability of the ankle joint.[32] With 1 mm depth, the group created different defect sizes at the talus. The area defect sizes are 2×2 mm^2, 4×4 mm^2, 6×6 mm^2, 8×8 mm^2, 10×10 mm^2, and 12×12 mm^2. In each group, the finite element method was used to simulate the stress on the ankle joint in the push-off phase, the midstance phase, and heel-strike phase to determine the contact pressure on the joint surface. The stress, contact state, and displacement of each component

changes while CT is more accurate in assessing the shape and dimensions of the lesion, not being able to inform about the involvement of the bone marrow. Each imaging examination has its virtues and defects, so we recommend a judicious combination to reach an accurate diagnosis.

of the ankle joint were observed in the different groups to determine its maximum value and location. Authors did not find significant changes when defect size was smaller than 6×6 mm^2, and stress reached the highest level in midstance phase and push-off phases when the defect size was 12×12 mm^2.

The reduction of joint contact area results in the increase of the intra-articular stresses. Ramsey and Hamilton concluded that a 42% reduction in the average contact area of ankle joints was found when the talus displaced laterally for 1 mm.[33] Increase in the defect size triggered higher mechanical stress in damaged talar cartilage and vice versa. Recent study created a finite element model based on CT images of ankle joint to simulate different defect sizes and stress forces throughout ankle movement.[34] Authors found that, regardless of direction of ankle movement, the peak stress on the talar carti-lage increased as the size of the defect region expanded and the peak stress of the defect size 2 cm^2 doubles the peak magnitude of the defect size 0.5 cm^2 in any ankle movements except for eversion. They also observed that the peak stresses of talar cartilage mostly appeared in the surrounding area of the defected cartilage.

In an attempt to resolve the lack of information on the relationship between the size of osteochondral lesions of the talus and their prognosis after treatment using the BMS technique, Ramponi and colleagues performed a meta-analysis that gathered the re-sults of 1868 ankles treated with this method.[35] The mean area was 103.8 ± 10.2 mm^2 in 20 studies, and the mean diameter was 10.0 ± 3.2 mm in 5 studies. Correlation with lesion area and diameter was heterogeneous, some of them positive correlated poorer outcomes with area and diameter, and some did not. Despite this, the statistical eval-uation allowed authors to conclude that OLT with areas greater than 107.4 mm^2, which corresponds to a maximum diameter of 10.2 mm, are significantly correlated with worse clinical results.

It is currently accepted that debridement, curettage, and BMS can be considered in lesions presenting a diameter less than 10 mm, with surface area less than 100 mm^2 and a depth less than 5 mm.[36] As such that surface area greater than 150 mm^2, overall osteochondral lesion depth greater than 7.8 mm, smoking history, age over 40 years, and uncontained lesions are factors that contribute to poor results.

SUMMARY

OLT is the most frequent cause of chronic ankle pain after traumatic episodes of the ankle, such as ankle sprain and fracture. Because ankle sprain is the most frequent sport lesion, OLT is more frequent in men in their 30s. These lesions can cause great impact in patient's quality of life, with a decrease in motor psychological function as high as patients presenting with lumbar sciatic pain. Lesions are more frequently located centromedial, representing up to two-thirds of all other sites. Size is one of the most relevant predictors of poor outcome. It is currently considered that OLT of up to 100 mm^2 can behave in a more indolent condition and can be either treated nonoperative or with BMS with good results. Above that area, the defect tends to transmit more shearing forces to adjacent cartilage and is more symptomatic. A broad discussion on how to address defects greater than 150 mm^2 is still in debate.

CLINICS CARE POINTS

- OLT is highly associated to CAI. Traumatic insult has been related to 93% to 98% of lateral defects and 61% to 70% of medial defects.

- Two-thirds of the lesions were located on the medial part of the talus (73%), 28% in the posteromedial (zone 7), and 31% centromedial (zone 4). Together, all lateral lesions sum up to 24%, and central lesions only 5%.
- Medial OLT present a mean size of 104 mm^2 (92–104 mm), whereas lateral lesions tend to be wider (92–154 mm^2), and central ones even wider (134–205 mm^2).
- Ankle radiographic images can fail to detect up to 30% to 46% of OLT. Currently, either or MRI or CT can be chosen to study lesion's size and site.
- The size of the lesion may have an effect on patient outcomes because larger lesions can alter the contact stresses of the ankle joint.
- OLT with surface area less than 100 mm^2 and a depth less than 5 mm present good results when treated with debridement, curettage, and BMS.

DISCLOSURE

The Authors have nothing to disclose.

REFERENCES

1. Murawski CD, Jamal MS, Hurley ET, et al. Terminology for osteochondral lesions of the ankle: proceedings of the International Consensus Meeting on Cartilage Repair of the Ankle. J ISAKOS 2022;7(2):62–6.
2. van Diepen PR, Dahmen J, Altink JN, et al. Location Distribution of 2,087 Osteochondral Lesions of the Talus. Cartilage 2021;13(1_suppl):1344S–53S.
3. König F. Veber freie Körper in der Gelenken. Dtsch. Z. Chir. 1888;27:90–109.
4. Kappis M. Weitere Beitrage zur traumatisch-mechanischen Entstehung der "spontanen" Knorpelablosungen. Deutsch Z Chir 1922;171:13–29.
5. van Dijk CN, Reilingh ML, Zengerink M, et al. Osteochondral defects in the ankle: Why painful? Knee Surgery. Sport Traumatol Arthrosc 2010;18(5):570–80.
6. Schachter AK, Chen AL, Reddy PD, et al. Osteochondral lesions of the talus. J Am Acad Orthop Surg 2005;13:152–8.
7. Frenkel SR, Di Cesare PE. Degradation and repair of articular cartilage. Front Biosci 1999;4:671–85.
8. Verhagen RA, Struijs PA, Bossuyt PM, et al. Systematic review of treatment strategies for osteochondral defects of the talar dome. Foot Ankle Clin 2003;8: 233–42.
9. Soboroff SH, Pappius EM, Komaroff AL. Benefits, risks, and costs of alternative approaches to the evaluation and treatment of severe ankle sprain. Clin Orthop Relat Res 1984;183:160–8.
10. Yeung M, Chan KM, So C, et al. An epidemiological survey on ankle sprain. Br J Sports Med 1994;28(2):112–6.
11. Savage-Elliott I, Ross KA, Smyth NA, et al. Osteochondral Lesions of the Talus: A Current Concepts Review and Evidence-Based Treatment Paradigm. Foot Ankle Spec 2014;7(5):414–22.
12. Bae S, Lee HK, Lee K, et al. Comparison of Arthroscopic and Magnetic Resonance Imaging Findings in Osteochondral Lesions of the Talus. Foot Ankle Int 2012;33(12):1058–62.
13. Deng E, Gao L, Shi W, et al. Both Magnetic Resonance Imaging and Computed Tomography Are Reliable and Valid in Evaluating Cystic Osteochondral Lesions of the Talus. Orthop J Sport Med 2020;8(9):1–7.

14. Krause F, Anwander H. Osteochondral lesion of the talus: still a problem? EFORT Open Rev 2022;7(6):337–43.
15. Zengerink M, Szerb I, Hangody L, et al. Current Concepts: Treatment of Osteochondral Ankle Defects. Foot Ankle Clin 2006;11(2):331–59.
16. D'Ambrosi R, Maccario C, Serra N, et al. Relationship between symptomatic osteochondral lesions of the talus and quality of life, body mass index, age, size and anatomic location. Foot Ankle Surg 2018;24(4):365–72.
17. Kodraliu G, Mosconi P, Groth N, et al. Subjective health status assessment: evaluation of the Italian version of the SF- 12 Health Survey: Results from the MiOS Project. J Epidemiol Biostat 2001;6:305–16.
18. Seo SG, Kim JS, Seo DK, et al. Osteochondral lesions of the talus: Few patients require surgery. Acta Orthop 2018;89(4):462–7.
19. Berndt AI, Harty M. Transchondral fractures (osteochondritis dissecans) of the talus. J Bone Joint Surg Am 1959 Sep;41-A:988–1020.
20. Raikin SM, Elias I, Zoga AC, et al. Osteochondral Lesions of the Talus: Localization and Morphologic Data from 424 Patients Using a Novel Anatomical Grid Scheme. Foot Ankle Int 2007;28(2):154–61.
21. Nakasa T, Ikuta Y, Sawa M, et al. Relationship Between Bone Marrow Lesions on MRI and Cartilage Degeneration in Osteochondral Lesions of the Talar Dome. Foot Ankle Int 2018;39(8):908–15.
22. Choi WJ, Park KK, Kim BS, et al. Osteochondral lesion of the talus: Is There a critical defect size for poor outcome? Am J Sports Med 2009;37(10):1974–80.
23. Valderrabano V. In: Valderrabano V, Easley M, editors. Foot and ankle sports orthopaedics. Cham: Springer International Publishing; 2016.
24. Flick AB, Gould N. Osteochondritis dissecans of the talus: review of the literature and new surgical approach for medial lesions. Foot Ankle 1985;5:165–85.
25. Mintz DN, Tashjian GS, Connell DA, et al. Osteochondral lesions of the talus: A new magnetic resonance grading system with arthroscopic correlation. J Arthrosc Relat Surg. 2003;19(4):353–9.
26. Tamam C, Tamam MO, Yildirim D, et al. Diagnostic value of single-photon emission computed tomography combined with computed tomography in relation to MRI on osteochondral lesions of the talus. Nucl Med Commun 2015;36:808–14.
27. Hepple S, Winson IG, Glew D. Osteochondral Lesions of the Talus: A Revised Classification. Foot Ankle Int 1999;20(12):789–93.
28. Nakasa T, Adachi N, Kato T, et al. Appearance of subchondral bone in computed tomography is related to cartilage damage in osteochondral lesions of the talar dome. Foot Ankle Int 2014;35(6):600–6.
29. Buckwalter JA, Mankin HJ. Articular cartilage: degeneration and osteoarthritis, repair, regeneration, and transplantation. Instr Course Lect 1998;47:487–504.
30. Chuckpaiwong B, Berkson EM, Theodore GH. Microfracture for Osteochondral Lesions of the Ankle: Outcome Analysis and Outcome Predictors of 105 Cases. Arthrosc J Arthrosc Relat Surg 2008;24(1):106–12.
31. Cuttica DJ, Smith WB, Hyer CF, et al. Osteochondral lesions of the talus: Predictors of clinical outcome. Foot Ankle Int 2011;32(11):1045–51.
32. Li J, Wang Y, Wei Y, et al. The effect of talus osteochondral defects of different area size on ankle joint stability: a finite element analysis. BMC Musculoskelet Disord 2022;23(1):1–10.
33. Ramsey PL, Hamilton W. Changes in tibiotalar area of contact caused by lateral talar shift. J Bone Joint Surg Am 1976;58(3):356–7.

34. Ruan Y, Du Y, Jiang Z, et al. The Biomechanical Influence of Defected Cartilage on the Progression of Osteochondral Lesions of the Talus: A Three-dimensional Finite Element Analysis. Orthop Surg 2023;April:1–9.

35. Ramponi L, Yasui Y, Murawski CD, et al. Lesion Size Is a Predictor of Clinical Outcomes after Bone Marrow Stimulation for Osteochondral Lesions of the Talus: A Systematic Review. Am J Sports Med 2017;45(7):1698–705.

36. Powers RT, Dowd TC, Giza E. Surgical Treatment for Osteochondral Lesions of the Talus. Arthroscopy 2021;37(12):3393–6.

Subtalar Osteochondral Lesions
Diagnosis, Indications, and Prognosis

Allison L. Boden, MD[a], Jonathan Kaplan, MD[b],
Amiethab Aiyer, MD[c],*

KEYWORDS

- Osteochondral lesion • Osteochondritis dissecans • Subtalar joint • Cartilage injury
- Calcaneus • Posterior facet • Foot and ankle

KEY POINTS

- Osteochondral lesions of the subtalar joint can occur with both high- and low-energy trauma.
- When plain radiographs are nondiagnostic, computerized tomography and MRI can aid in the diagnosis of subtalar osteochondral lesions.
- There is a paucity of literature on subtalar osteochondral lesions, including prevalence, treatment options, and prognosis/outcomes.

INTRODUCTION

An osteochondral lesion (OCL) is an injury that involves damage to both the bone and the cartilage.[1,2] Many terms have been used to refer to this clinically, including osteochondritis dissecans (OCD), osteochondral fracture, and osteochondral defect.[2] The most frequent anatomic locations for an OCL include the knee, elbow, and talar dome.[1] Less frequently, OCLs can occur in the subtalar joint. Historically, OCLs of the subtalar joint were thought to occur with high-energy trauma like subtalar dislocation or calcaneus fracture; however, there is literature supporting the presence of OCLs of the subtalar joint with low-energy trauma or no history of trauma at all.[2,3]

The subtalar joint is a complex joint that is responsible for hindfoot inversion and eversion.[4–6] It includes the talocalcaneal and talonavicular joints.[4–6] The superior articular surface of the calcaneus consists of 3 facets that make up the subtalar joint: the

[a] Department of Orthopedic Surgery, Hospital for Special Surgery, 535 East 70th Street, New York, NY 10021, USA; [b] Department of Orthopedic Surgery, Duke University, 1816 Hillandale Road, Durham, NC 27705, USA; [c] Department of Orthopedic Surgery, Johns Hopkins University, 4940 Eastern Avenue, Baltimore, MD 21244, USA
* Corresponding author.
E-mail address: tabsaiyer@gmail.com

Foot Ankle Clin N Am 29 (2024) 225–233
https://doi.org/10.1016/j.fcl.2023.07.002
1083-7515/24/© 2023 Elsevier Inc. All rights reserved.

anterior, middle, and posterior facets.[4–6] The posterior facet is the largest facet of the 3 and is the main weightbearing surface of the talocalcaneal joint.[4–6] It is separated from the anterior and middle facets by the sinus tarsi and tarsal canal.[4–6]

Identification of subtalar pathology can be difficult due to the complexity of the joint and need for advanced imaging.

PRESENTATION

The first step in assessing ankle or hindfoot pain is to perform a thorough history and physical examination. Patients with subtalar OCLs often present similarly to patients with OCLs of the talar dome and separating tibio-talar pathology from talo-calcaneal pathology can sometimes be challenging (**Box 1**). The most common mechanism of injury for a subtalar osteochondral injury is an inversion/eversion injury to the foot/ankle, and patients are often misdiagnosed as having an ankle or subtalar sprain. Patients typically report a progressive, deep, dull aching pain at the ankle or lateral hindfoot. The pain is often aggravated by strenuous activity and weightbearing and improved with rest. Mechanical symptoms, including locking and catching, are rarely the chief complaint; however, the feeling of instability when walking on uneven surfaces is common. Patients often report difficulty with ambulation and may have an antalgic gait. In a patient with ankle pain after minimal or no trauma or a patient with chronic ankle pain after resolution of an acute injury, osteochondral injury should remain on the differential diagnosis list.

In patients with an acute injury, the ankle and foot are often diffusely edematous and painful, which can limit the specificity of the physical examination. On examination, patients typically have tenderness to palpation at the lateral aspect of the subtalar joint and sinus tarsi and often have limited range of motion of the subtalar joint. An injury to the subtalar joint should be suspected in a patient with persistent edema, difficulty with weightbearing, and loss of subtalar motion.

DIAGNOSIS

Although the presence of an OCL on the talar dome is occasionally apparent on X-ray, diagnosis of OCLs in the subtalar joint can sometimes prove to be more difficult. When patients present with foot or ankle-related pain, initial evaluation after history and physical examination is generally with plain radiographs to assess for fracture or other pathology. Anteroposterior, lateral, and oblique radiographs of the foot and ankle may be nondiagnostic or may show a radiolucent region at the posterior, medial, or lateral process of the talus indicating a possible OCL (**Fig. 1**).[1]

Box 1
Common symptoms of subtalar osteochondral lesion

Dull, aching hindfoot pain

Edema

Worse with activity

Better with rest

Unstable or "giving way"

Locking/catching

Difficulty with ambulation

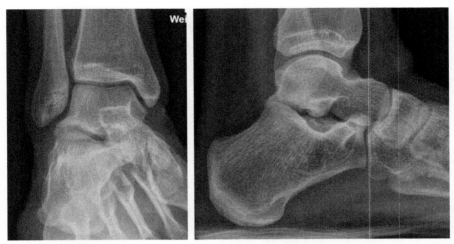

Fig. 1. AP and lateral radiographs of a right ankle demonstrate a subtalar osteochondral lesion.

If plain radiographs (XR) are nondiagnostic, advanced imaging with a computerized tomography (CT) scan or MRI can be obtained to better evaluate the subtalar joint.[1,7] Both CT and MRI have improved the sensitivity and specificity of diagnosis and characterization of osteochondral injuries.[7] Classic imaging findings on CT scan include subchondral fracture or fragmentation, subchondral cysts, sclerosis, loose bodies, or osteoarthritic changes.[1] Classic imaging findings on MRI include a well-defined hypointense signal on T1 with adjacent bone marrow edema (**Fig. 2**).[1] Additional findings may include a joint effusion, loose bodies, subchondral cysts, or other evidence of osteoarthritic changes (**Box 2**).[1] Regardless of whether the plain radiographs demonstrate an OCL, advanced imaging may be helpful to demonstrate the location, size, and depth of the lesion.[7] Additionally, MRI can assess the overlying articular cartilage, subchondral edema, and stability of the lesion. Subtalar lidocaine or corticosteroid injection can also function as both a therapeutic and diagnostic treatment modality.

In the setting of subtalar pathology without obvious OCL on advanced imaging, evaluation with subtalar arthroscopy can be performed. In comparison to CT and MRI, arthroscopy has the advantage of direct visualization of the joint and can provide both diagnostic and therapeutic value. Diagnostic subtalar arthroscopy is indicated for patients with persistent pain, edema, stiffness, locking, or catching that is resistant to conservative management.[8,9]

INDICATIONS

Like treatment of OCLs of the talar dome, surgical treatment for OCLs of the subtalar joint is typically reserved for patients who fail conservative management. Nonsurgical management includes the use of nonsteroidal anti-inflammatory medications (NSAIDs), immobilization, non-weightbearing for 4 to 6 weeks, and then physical therapy.[2,10]

When conservative measures fail, surgical treatment is then considered. Unfortunately, there is a paucity of literature that exists specifically investigating the treatment of subtalar OCD; however, in the existing literature, most surgeons use the same

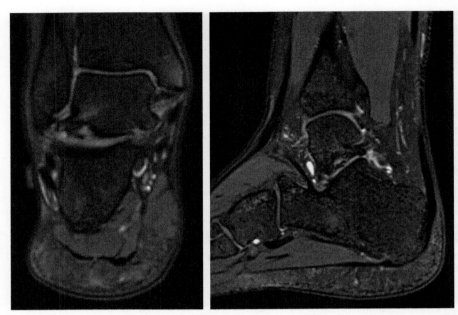

Fig. 2. Coronal and sagittal MR images of a right ankle in a patient with an osteochondral lesion in the subtalar joint. There is evidence of subchondral fracture and fragmentation.

principles used to treat OCLs of the talar dome. Surgery is often performed arthroscopically but sometimes necessitates a mini-arthrotomy to access the OCL.[9,11,12] As detailed in the current evidence section below, the mainstay of treatment is osteochondral excision and curettage with additional intervention including possible microfracture, drilling, or bone grafting and fixation. If there are significant secondary arthritic changes noted at the subtalar joint, arthrodesis may be a reasonable treatment option.[3]

CURRENT EVIDENCE

Although there is a large amount of literature published on the diagnosis, management, and outcomes of OCLs of the talar dome, a paucity of literature exists for OCLs of the subtalar joint. To our knowledge there have been only 5 case reports published in the last 30 years that discuss OCLs or OCD of the subtalar joint and 2

Box 2
Classic MRI findings of subtalar osteochondral lesion

Hypointense lesion on T1

Subchondral edema

Joint effusion

Subtalar loose body

Subchondral cyst

Subtalar arthritic changes

of which are in the pediatric age group (**Table 1**).[11–15] We will summarize the case reports and the minimal other literature published on OCLs of the subtalar joint to highlight not only the typical presentation, but also the variety of treatment options and algorithms used.

One of the first case reports was published in 2005 by Madi and colleagues,[14] who reported on a case of OCD of the subtalar facet in a 10 year old male with no history of trauma. The patient complained of ankle pain and stiffness for several weeks.[14] On examination there was no evidence of edema, but the patient did have decreased range of motion of the subtalar joint.[14] Radiographs and CT showed an OCL of the subtalar joint.[14] The patient was treated conservatively with immobilization in a non-weightbearing short leg cast for 6 weeks.[14] Last follow-up was at 6 months and at that time the patient had no residual symptoms and had resumed all previous activities.[14]

Kadakia and colleagues also treated an OCL of the subtalar joint in a pediatric patient; however, this patient was treated operatively.[11] In contrast to the acute presentation in the Madi and colleagues case, this 14 year old female presented with a 3 year history of hindfoot pain and the inability to perform strenuous activity or sports. On examination, the patient's gait was antalgic, and she had significantly diminished subtalar range of motion.[11] Radiographs were negative, so a CT scan was obtained that demonstrated a 0.5 cm subtalar OCD in the lateral aspect of the posterior facet and a loose body within the subtalar joint.[11] A trial of NSAIDs and 4 weeks in a non-weightbearing short leg cast was initially successful; however, symptoms recurred within 2 weeks of cast removal.[11] With recurrence of the symptoms, a subtalar injection was performed that lead to complete resolution of symptoms for 1 hour.[11] Continuation of NSAIDs and use of a removable boot lead to improvement of the symptoms after roughly 6 weeks and physical therapy was then initiated.[11] Recurrence of the symptoms occurred again and at that time the patient was taken to the operating room for arthroscopy to evaluate the subtalar joint.[11] The OCD was identified and a miniarthrotomy was used to gain access to the OCD lesion, after which the lesion was excised, and curettage and drilling were performed.[11] The patient was back to all activities by 3 months postoperatively and at her 1-year follow-up, she continued to have complete resolution of symptoms.[11]

The treatment of OCD in adults tends to follow a similar pattern in which patients are treated operatively only after conservative treatment has failed to improve symptoms. Cugat and colleagues[13] reported a 34 year old male in Spain with pain in the tarsal canal area when ambulating and standing who failed conservative management of rest and NSAIDs. Plain radiographs were normal; however, a scintographic imaging study showed hypersignal in the symptomatic area.[13] MRI confirmed the presence of an OCL of the subtalar joint.[13] Arthroscopic debridement was performed, which improved the patients pain and function.[13] At 24 months postoperatively, the patient remained asymptomatic and was back to work.[13]

Despite continued improvements in advanced imaging, there remain times that CT and MRI fail to diagnose an OCL and the lesion is discovered intraoperatively. Moonot and colleagues[12] treated a 34 year old male laborer who had a twisting injury to his ankle 2 years prior that was treated as an ankle sprain. However, the patient continued to have pain aggravated by activity and alleviated with rest.[12] The patient also described locking episodes.[12] On examination, the patient had tenderness to palpation along the sinus tarsi, but his range of motion was relatively symmetric to his contralateral foot and ankle.[12] Plain radiographs and MRI showed arthritic changes in the subtalar joint, a subchondral cystic lesion, and loose bodies within the subtalar joint.[12] Given the failure of conservative management, the decision was made to

Table 1
Summary of published case reports

Study	Patient Age/Gender	Lesion Size	Operative?	Loose Body?	Treatment Details
Madi et al,[14] 2005	10 M	-	No	No	Non-weightbearing (NWB), short leg cast 6 wk
Kadakia & Sarkar,[11] 2007	14 F	0.5 cm	Yes	Yes	NSAIDs, NWB, short leg cast 4 wk → Injection, removable boot, physical therapy (PT) → Mini-arthrotomy with excision, curettage, drilling
Cugat et al,[13] 2007	34 M	-	Yes	No	NSAIDs, rest → Arthroscopic debridement
Moonot & Sharma,[12] 2021	34 M	1.2 × 1.5 cm	Yes	Yes	Mini-arthrotomy, excision, debridement, autograft and open reduction with internal fixation (ORIF)
Yanagisawa et al,[15] 2021	24 M	-	L: No R: Yes	L: No R: Yes	L: ankle taping, activity modification R: injection → arthroscopic removal of loose bodies

proceed with surgical debridement of the subchondral cyst.[12] A miniopen 3 cm incision was used to examine the subtalar joint and a previously unidentified OCL was identified.[12] The OCL was removed to debride and curettage the underlying subchondral cyst and the loose bodies were removed.[12] Next, autograft from the ipsilateral calcaneus was used to fill the defect and the osteochondral fragment was fixed using a 4 mm partially threaded cannulated cancellous screw.[12] The patient was immobilized for 2 weeks and kept non-weightbearing for 6 weeks.[12] At the 1 year follow-up visit, the patient had returned to all prior activities, had no recurrence of symptoms, and postoperative CT scan showed full bony consolidation at the operative site.[12] Additionally, the patient's foot and ankle disability score improved from 26.0 to 92.3 at the 1 year follow-up visit.[12]

OCLs in the subtalar joint can occur bilaterally. Yanagisawa and colleagues[15] published the first case report documenting the presence and treatment of bilateral subtalar OCDs, which occurred in a 24 year old professional soccer player. This patient began to experience insidious onset of left hindfoot pain at the age of 16 years.[15] Radiographs were normal; however, CT and MRI were consistent with an OCL.[15] He was treated with ankle taping and activity modification and the pain resolved after 3 months.[15] He was able to return to his full training program without symptom recurrence.[15] Four years later at the age of 20 years, the patient experienced similar symptoms in the right hindfoot with no obvious traumatic event.[15] Similarly to the contralateral side, a CT and MRI showed an OCL, but in addition there were 2 loose bodies identified on imaging.[15] A subtalar lidocaine injection completely resolved the pain and the patient was able to continue training for soccer, though the symptoms recurred.[15] He subsequently underwent removal of loose bodies, but no microfracture of the OCL was performed.[15] He was able to return to training 2 weeks after the surgery and returned to professional games 6 months postoperatively.[15] The player remained symptom free 4 years from surgery and continued to play professional soccer.[15]

Consistent with the above case reports, OCLs can be found in patients without a history of high-energy trauma. Choi and colleagues[3] reported 10 patients who had osteochondral fractures of the subtalar joint without history of dislocation. In this study (and consistent with the published nonpediatric case reports), the average age of the patient was 25 years (range 19–32) and all patients had a history of a fall or twisting injury to their foot 6 to 24 months prior to evaluation by the authors.[3] All patients complained of pain in the subtalar region and 70% had lost the majority of their subtalar motion.[3] Plain radiographs were obtained and compared to initial XRs and either CT or MRI was obtained to evaluate for subtalar pathology. Osteochondral injury was confined to the posterior facet in 7 patients, both the anterior and posterior facets in one case, and the sustentaculum tali in one case.[3] Seventy percent of patients were noted to have degenerative changes of the subtalar joint.[3] Six patients were treated with subtalar fusion, 1 patient with a triple arthrodesis, and 3 with physical therapy.[3] Seven out of 8 patients who underwent fusion reported no pain at follow-up.[3] One patient who underwent fusion and all 3 patients who had physical therapy reported mild pain at follow-up.[3] The authors concluded that if motion can be preserved, a reasonable functional outcome is possible; however, if motion is lost, an arthrodesis can produce satisfactory results.[3]

Osteochondral injury to the subtalar joint is probably more prevalent than the literature indicates. A study by Angthong and colleagues[16] in 2019 reported the prevalence of OCLs of the subtalar joint following intra-articular calcaneus fracture. Of the 30 patients analyzed in the study, 28 patients (93.3%) were found to have OCLs of the subtalar joint on CT mapping.[16] Most of the lesions were at the anterior (57.1%)

or central (46.4%) aspect of the posterior facet.[16] Severity of calcaneus fracture (Sanders grade) showed a trend toward a higher prevalence of OCLs (P = .181).[16] Interestingly, the authors found no statistically significant relationship between the presence of an OCL and osteoarthritic changes in follow-up radiographs.[16] The authors concluded that the prevalence of OCLs of the subtalar joint is high in the presence of intra-articular calcaneus fractures.[16]

PROGNOSIS

In all previously discussed publications, the patients did well and were asymptomatic at final follow-up, which ranged from 6 months to 4 years. Unfortunately, there is not enough high-level evidence on OCLs of the subtalar joint to make any strong prognostic claims, especially because all published studies are small.

Despite the lack of literature on subtalar OCD outcomes, there is some evidence that treatment of subtalar pathology with arthroscopy leads to improved outcomes. Ahn and colleagues[17] evaluated the clinical outcomes of 115 consecutive patients with a variety of conditions who were treated with subtalar arthroscopy from November 2002 to April 2008 with at least 1 year of follow-up (average 48 months). All patients had failed conservative management, including NSAIDs, physical therapy, shoe modification, and injection, for a minimum of 3 months.[17] Six patients in this study had OCLs of the subtalar joint and underwent excision and drilling.[17] Within the study, a clinical rating scale was used to measure outcomes and 59% of patients reported excellent, 38% reported good, and 3% reported poor outcomes.[17] It is important to note that none of the 6 patients treated for OCL of the subtalar joint reported their outcomes as poor. This study provides some evidence that patient with OCLs of the subtalar joint can have reasonable outcomes with arthroscopic excision and drilling; however, like the previous studies mentioned, the study size was small.

CLINICS CARE POINTS

- An injury to the subtalar joint should be suspected in a patient with significant swelling, difficulty with weightbearing, and subtalar joint stiffness.
- If plain radiographs are negative, patients should obtain a CT or MRI scan to better evaluate for subtalar pathology.
- The incidence and prevalence of subtalar osteochondral injury may be grossly underestimated.

FUTURE DIRECTIONS

Given there is a paucity of literature on the ideal treatment algorithm and both operative and nonoperative outcomes, more research is needed to gain better clarity on surgical indications and outcomes of various treatment options.

DISCLOSURES

The authors have no relevant relationships to disclose.

REFERENCES

1. Sanders RK, Crim JR. Osteochondral injuries. Semin Ultrasound CT MR 2001; 22(4):352–70.

2. Badekas T, Takvorian M, Souras N. Treatment principles for osteochondral lesions in foot and ankle. Int Orthop 2013;37(9):1697–706.
3. Choi CH, Ogilvie-Harris DJ. Occult osteochondral fractures of the subtalar joint: a review of 10 patients. J Foot Ankle Surg 2002;41(1):40–3.
4. Barg A, Tochigi Y, Amendola A, et al. Subtalar instability: diagnosis and treatment. Foot Ankle Int 2012;33(2):151–60.
5. Krahenbuhl N, Horn-Lang T, Hintermann B, et al. The subtalar joint: A complex mechanism. EFORT Open Rev 2017;2(7):309–16.
6. Rockar PA Jr. The subtalar joint: anatomy and joint motion. J Orthop Sports Phys Ther 1995;21(6):361–72.
7. Verhagen RA, Maas M, Dijkgraaf MG, et al. Prospective study on diagnostic strategies in osteochondral lesions of the talus. Is MRI superior to helical CT? J Bone Joint Surg Br 2005;87(1):41–6.
8. Siddiqui MA, Chong KW, Yeo W, et al. Subtalar arthroscopy using a 2.4-mm zero-degree arthroscope: indication, technical experience, and results. Foot Ankle Spec 2010;3(4):167–71.
9. Hsu AR, Gross CE, Lee S, et al. Extended indications for foot and ankle arthroscopy. J Am Acad Orthop Surg 2014;22(1):10–9.
10. Powell BD, Cooper MT. Ankle MRI and Arthroscopy Correlation With Cartilaginous Defects and Symptomatic Os Trigonum. Sports Med Arthrosc Rev 2017;25(4):237–45.
11. Kadakia AP, Sarkar J. Osteochondritis dissecans of the talus involving the subtalar joint: a case report. J Foot Ankle Surg 2007;46(6):488–92.
12. Moonot P, Sharma G. Osteochondritis Dissecans of the Lateral Process of Talus Involving the Subtalar Joint: An Unusual Case. J Foot Ankle Surg 2021;60(3):630–3.
13. Cugat R, Cusco X, Garcia M, et al. Posterosuperior osteochondritis of the calcaneus. Arthroscopy 2007;23(9). 1025 e1021-1024.
14. Madi F, Vialle R, Mary P, et al. Osteochondritis dissecans of the subtalar articular facet: an unusual diagnosis. Pediatr Radiol 2005;35(8):823–5.
15. Yanagisawa Y, Ishii T, Yamazaki M. Bilateral Osteochondritis Dissecans of the Talar Posterior Calcaneal Articular Surface in a Professional Soccer Player: A Case Report. J Orthop Case Rep 2021;11(3):55–8.
16. Angthong C, Veljkovic A, Angthong W, et al. Talar-sided osteochondral lesion of the subtalar joint following the intra-articular calcaneal fracture: study via a modified computed tomography mapping analysis. Eur J Orthop Surg Traumatol 2019;29(6):1331–6.
17. Ahn JH, Lee SK, Kim KJ, et al. Subtalar arthroscopic procedures for the treatment of subtalar pathologic conditions: 115 consecutive cases. Orthopedics 2009;32(12):891.

Preoperative and Postoperative Imaging and Outcome Scores for Osteochondral Lesion Repair of the Ankle

Loek D. Loozen, MD, PhD[a,b,*], Alastair S. Younger, MD, FRCSC[a,b],
Andrea N. Veljkovic, MD, FRCSC, MPH, Bcomm[a,b,c]

KEYWORDS

• Osteochondral lesion • Ankle joint • Imaging • MRI • Cartilage imaging

KEY POINTS

• The utilization of more than four distinct patient-reported outcome scores to evaluate treatment efficacy introduces a lack of standardization, impeding the conduct of comparative research.

• During the preoperative stage, MRI has proven to be an indispensable noninvasive modality for the evaluation of alterations in articular cartilage and subchondral bone.

• Subsequent to cartilage repair, MRI offers valuable insights into tissue repair, defect filling percentage, and the integration of the repaired tissue with the subchondral bone.

INTRODUCTION

Symptomatic cartilage lesions in the ankle pose a significant challenge and often require surgical intervention to alleviate pain, improve joint function, and restore the integrity of the articular surface. These lesions frequently coincide with damage to the underlying bone, known as osteochondral lesions. In the ankle joint, these lesions are predominantly found on the talar dome, while the distal tibia is less susceptible to such injuries due to its mechanical and anatomic characteristics. Occasionally,

[a] Division of Distal Extremities, Department of Orthopaedics, University of British Columbia, Vancouver, British Columbia, Canada; [b] Footbridge Clinic for Integrated Orthopaedic Care, 221 Keefer Place, Vancouver, British Columbia, V6B 6C1, Canada; [c] University of British Columbia, Adult Foot and Ankle Reconstructive Surgery, Department of Orthopaedics, Vancouver, British Columbia, Canada
* Corresponding author. Footbridge Clinic for Integrated Orthopaedic Care, 3412 W 2nd Avenue, Vancouver, British Columbia V6R 1J2, Canada
E-mail address: loekloozen@gmail.com

Foot Ankle Clin N Am 29 (2024) 235–252
https://doi.org/10.1016/j.fcl.2023.11.003
1083-7515/24/© 2023 Elsevier Inc. All rights reserved.

osteochondral lesions may affect multiple bone articular surfaces, although this is rare. Among talar dome lesions, the majority, approximately 65% of cases, are located on the medial ridge. The second most common location is the lateral ridge, accounting for around 32% of cases. Lesions situated in the middle of the talar dome are relatively uncommon, constituting only about 3% of cases. There are also rare instances where osteochondral lesions occur on the distal fibula. It is worth noting that osteochondral lesions on the medial aspect of the talar dome tend to be larger in terms of surface area and depth compared to lesions on the lateral side.[1–3]

Bone marrow stimulation (BMS), consisting of lesion curettage and microfracture, is the most commonly performed procedure for managing symptomatic osteochondral lesions of the talus (OLTs).[4] Numerous studies have demonstrated excellent short-term and mid-term clinical outcomes with this technique. However, long-term deterioration of the reparative fibrocartilage has been reported in up to 35% of patients.[5,6] This progressive fibrocartilage deterioration may be attributed, at least in part, to persistent mechanical instability or underlying biological insufficiency. Therefore, a size limit of 15 mm in diameter has been recommended for BMS procedures.[7] In the management of larger defects, BMS is often supplemented with additional agents like biologics or scaffolds. Concentrated bone marrow aspirate and platelet-rich plasma are commonly used in conjunction with BMS to enhance the repair process.[7,8] Scaffolds include commercially available products often derived from allogeneic cartilage. Alongside these approaches, other treatment strategies have evolved, such as mosaicplasty (osteochondral autograft transfer system [OATS]), matrix-assisted autologous chondrocyte implantation [MACI], and autologous matrix-induced chondrogenesis (AMIC) (open AMIC and arthroscopic AMIC). The latter has gained popularity and has repeatedly shown good results at short-term to medium-term follow-up. Nevertheless, none of these strategies has proven superior as high-quality comparative studies are not available to date.[9,10] One of the main limiting factors is the lack of standardized outcome measurements and assessment modalities to evaluate the effectiveness of repair procedures.

The objective of this article is to present a comprehensive review of the current status of preoperative imaging of osteochondral defects of the ankle joint. The second part of the article focuses on examining the existing classification systems and patient-reported outcome measures (PROMs) used to evaluate the effectiveness of treatments. Furthermore, it aims to provide the latest information on radiological evaluation techniques for assessing the impact of cartilage repair.

IMAGING OF ANKLE CARTILAGE REPAIR

Conventional radiographs, although typically the first imaging approach used, may show positive but nonspecific findings, especially in chronic lesions, those with displacement, osteonecrosis, or cystic changes. They also have low sensitivity, particularly in acute nondisplaced lesions, and cannot assess the integrity of the articular cartilage surface. Loomer and colleagues[11] reported that 50% of OLTs are not detectable on plain radiographs. However, if there is an acute traumatic fracture involving the subchondral plate and cancellous subchondral bone, the fracture line may be visible on radiographs. As the lesion becomes chronic, various changes can occur locally. Central osteophyte formation, characterized by the growth of bony projections, may develop at the site of the chondral lesion. Additionally, subchondral cystic changes or the formation of areas of fluid-filled cavities, as well as sclerosis or increased bone density, can occur in the same region (**Fig. 1**). Osteophyte formation may also be observed at the margins of the joint, contributing to the overall presentation of

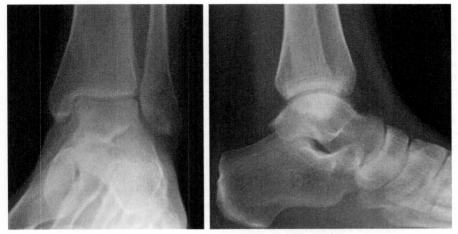

Fig. 1. Conventional imaging of osteochondral defect of medial talar dome in an 18-year-old female. Subchondral cystic changes and fluid-filled cavities are observed over the medial talar dome. Mild sclerosis and increased bone density are observed around the cysts.

the chondral lesion over time. These radiographic findings provide important insights into the chronicity and local effects of chondral lesions in the ankle and foot.[11,12]

Computed Tomography

Computed tomography (CT) scans provide detailed imaging of bony structures and can be useful for evaluating any changes in subchondral bone or the presence of osteophytes (**Fig. 2**). It's important to note that CT is not as effective as MRI in directly visualizing soft tissues, such as cartilage, compared to MRI. CT imaging offers a certain level of contrast resolution for soft tissues, as different tissue types can be distinguished based on Hounsfield units measurements. The use of newer dual-energy

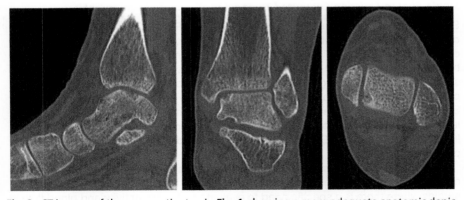

Fig. 2. CT images of the same patient as in **Fig. 1**, showing a more adequate anatomic depiction of the OLT. Subchondral cystic changes are observed with mild sclerosis and increased bone density are observed around the cysts. Cartilage thickness can be assessed indirectly by joint space but is not well visualized even in soft tissue setting (not depicted). CT, computed tomography; OLT, osteochondral lesion of the talus.

scanners further enhances soft tissue contrast.[13] In order to improve soft tissue resolution, intra-articular or intravenous contrast agents are often utilized to assess intra-articular structures. By employing CT with soft tissue kernel and postprocessing techniques, it is possible to identify areas of varying cartilage thickness, producing results comparable to MRI.[13] However, standard soft tissue CT imaging cannot effectively visualize the fine details of the cartilage necessary for early detection of cartilage change.

The utilization of contrast agents and specific acquisition methods has made it feasible to achieve cartilage details that correlate with MRI.[14] Typically, iodine-based contrast agents are commonly used during CT imaging, which are anionic in nature. The negatively charged glycosaminoglycans (GAGs) in the cartilage repel anionic agents. A key hallmark of cartilage damage and early osteoarthritis is the depletion of GAG content within the extracellular matrix.[15] As such, anionic contrast agents are concentrated in areas with low GAG content, such as synovial fluid or cartilage lesions, and excluded from regions that have a high density of GAGs, such as normal cartilage. This difference in contrast distribution can be detected accurately via CT.[16] The contrast-enhanced MRI technique, delayed gadolinium-enhanced MRI of cartilage (dGEMRIC), works in a similar fashion. In the aforementioned strategies, the contrast agent is administered intravenously. The contrast agent diffuses into the cartilage in a dose-dependent manner, inversely correlated with the fixed charged density of the cartilage, which is mainly composed of GAGs.[17,18]

Although the contrast-enhanced CT strategies have shown promise, they are primarily utilized in research settings and have not demonstrated clear advantages over conventional MRI thus far.[16] However, they may be considered as an alternative for evaluating cartilage in cases where patients experience claustrophobia during MRI examinations.

The use of plain radiographs, CT scans, and isotope bone scans in medical imaging exposes patients to ionizing radiation, which carries a risk of cancer induction and genetic damage. Although this risk is well established at high doses, its risk remains uncertain at low doses commonly used in medical imaging. Especially in children, to minimize this risk, MRI should be used whenever possible, particularly for follow-up imaging.[19]

Single-Photon Emission Computed Tomography/Computed Tomography

Single-photon emission computed tomography (SPECT)/CT provides valuable 3-dimensional (3D) localization of scintigraphic osteoblastic activity within the region of interest, offering supplementary information regarding the extent of subchondral bone involvement, vitality of the osteochondral lesion, and identification of multiple lesions. Meftah and colleagues[21] showed additional diagnostic value in preoperative planning by showing the precise location of the active segment in multiple lesions.[20,21] Small OLTs can be missed on MRI, which can be detected via SPECT/CT, and large lesions can have a low osteoblastic activity, and are not deemed symptomatic (**Fig. 3**). In about 5% of cases, SPECT/CT provides relevant additional information MRI has not provided.[22]

SPECT/CT is not commonly used as a routine imaging modality for assessing the quality of repaired cartilage. Its use is typically limited to specialized cases or research studies where there is a specific need to evaluate metabolic activity and blood flow in the repaired tissue. Therefore, SPECT/CT can determine if it resembles healthy, normal cartilage.[20,23,24] All in all, the authors recommend the use of SPECT/CT and MRI together for comprehensive diagnostic assessment of OLTs but see a limited role in the postoperative phase.

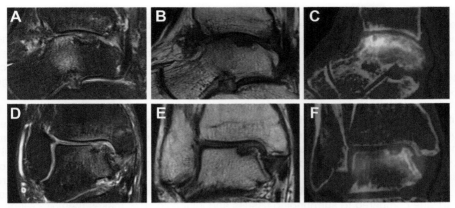

Fig. 3. MRI and SPECT/CT of a 50-year-old patient with an osteochondral lesion but at the same time cartilage degeneration through the anterior aspect of the ankle joint. The added value of SPECT is indicated: based on the sagittal images, the actual area with increased uptake appears more anterior than the actual osteochondral lesion which coincides with the bone edema on MRI, whereas the medial OLT has less uptake and little edema. (*A*) Sagittal T2. (*B*) Sagittal T1. (*C* and *F*) Sagittal and coronal SPECT/CT. (*D*) Coronal PD. (*E*) T2 FS. FS, fat suppression; OLT, osteochondral lesion of the talus; PD, proton density; SPECT/CT, single-photon emission computed tomography/computed tomography.

MRI

MRI has become an indispensable noninvasive method for assessing changes in articular cartilage and subchondral bone. Magnetic resonance (MR) examinations exhibit high diagnostic accuracy for OLTs, almost equal to arthroscopy with regard to the assessment of the cartilage.[25,26] With regard to the underlying bone and abnormalities, it is almost as good as CT.[18]

To diagnose osteochondral lesions with MRI, understanding the normal appearance of articular cartilage and bone tissue is crucial. On T1-weighted sequences, cartilage shows intermediate signal intensity, higher than muscle but lower than adipose tissue. Proton density (PD) sequences also display intermediate signal intensity for cartilage, between muscle and adipose tissue. However, on T2-weighted images, cartilage has a low signal intensity compared to the high signal intensity of adjacent synovial fluid, enabling accurate cartilage evaluation. Signal intensity of cartilage on T2-weighted images increases superficially. Cortical bone consistently exhibits low signal intensity on all MRI sequences, while medullary bone has high signal intensity on T1-weighted and T2-weighted images, reducing significantly on fat-saturated sequences.

Adjacent areas to osteochondral lesion fragments usually display intermediate or low signal intensity on T1-weighted images. The "rim sign," a distinct high signal line, is observable on T2-weighted images beside the fragment, indicating an unstable lesion.[27] Chondral defects can be identified on T2-weighted and PD sequences, exposing subchondral bone filled with synovial fluid, appearing as a high-intensity signal. Loose bodies appear as low signal areas surrounded by high signal fluid on T2 images. Subchondral cysts exhibit a high-intensity signal on T2-weighted and PD images but appear hypointense on T1-weighted images. Bone edema, commonly surrounding osteochondral lesions, shows low signal intensity on T1-weighted images and high signal intensity on T2-weighted fat-suppressed images or short tau inversion recovery sequences. MRI can differentiate between chronic and recent lesions, with low T1 signal intensity indicating sclerosis, a characteristic of chronic osteochondral lesions. **Table 1** presents the parameters of MRI assessment after cartilage repair, providing an overview of the specific MRI characteristics that are important to consider when evaluating the outcomes of these repair strategies (**Fig. 4**).

MRI sequences

Sequence protocols including 2-dimensional (2D) fast spin echo/turbo spin echo (FSE/TSE) are the most commonly used for clinical assessment of cartilage lesions as part of the International Cartilage Repair Society (ICRS)–recommended cartilage imaging protocol; T1-weighted, T2-weighted, PD-weighted, and intermediate-weighted sequences with or without fat suppression are available. The FSE and TSE protocols provide excellent signal-to-noise ratio, tissue contrast, and relatively fast acquisition times (**Table 2**).

Gradient recalled echo (GRE) imaging techniques provide high signal intensity for cartilage compared to surrounding tissues and joint fluid. This makes them excellent for segmenting and quantifying cartilage volume and thickness. However, susceptibility artifacts can be problematic at cartilage repair sites, and they are not sensitive to bone marrow lesions. Additionally, they are not suitable for detecting subtle focal cartilage defects. When susceptibility artifacts are not present, GRE can be used to quantify cartilage thickness and volume, including cartilage repair. However, it is not recommended for assessing focal cartilage defects or bone marrow edemalike lesions.[27]

Three-dimensional and compositional magnetic resonance techniques

Three-dimensional MRI sequences enable multiplanar reconstruction in all planes, regardless of the sequence acquisition plane. This capability reduces volume averaging effects, similar to thin-slice CT reconstructions, and provides higher resolution images in any plane. This is particularly useful for detecting thin abnormalities like fissures, especially on curved surfaces around the ankle. MRI visualization of oblique and curved structures is excellent with these techniques (see **Figs. 4** and **5**). Accurate detection and characterization of shallow, low-grade partial, and small articular cartilage defects pose challenges for any technique, but high–spatial resolution 3D MRI techniques perform exceptionally well in these cases.[28,29] There is a lack of high-quality comparative research comparing 2D and 3D MRI for assessing cartilage damage in the ankle joint. When comparing multiple novel 3D MRI techniques only

Table 1	
Parameters of MRI assessment after repair	
BMS, MACI, biomaterial matrix ± BMS.	Osteochondral allograft or autograft, mosaicplasty, OATS
Degree of filling of defect	Degree of filling of defect by transplanted osteochondral plugs
Morphologic characteristics of reparative tissue	Restoration of radial curvature of joint surface
Presence or absence of delamination	Presence or absence of displacement
Extent of peripheral integration (presence of fissures)	Peripheral integration of repair cartilage and osseous components
Morphologic characteristics of the repair site	Integrity of host cartilage

Abbreviations: BMS, bone marrow stimulation/microfracturing; MACI, matrix-assisted autologous chondrocyte implantation; OATS, osteochondral autograft transfer system.

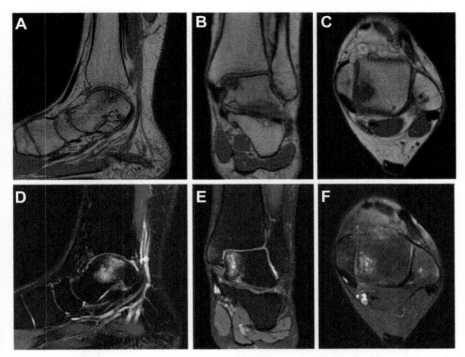

Fig. 4. MRI of the same patient as **Figs. 1** and **2**: 3D imaging with PD provides good visibility of cartilage on the talar dome as well as distal tibia (*A*). With high anatomic accuracy, suppression of the edema is observed in (*D–F*). The same for reconstructions in the coronal and axial planes (*B* & *C*). Bone edema can be well assessed on STIR images (*D*) which is often correlated with clinical symptoms. Fat-suppressed images provide extra information with regard to soft tissues around the ankle joint (*E* & *F*). (*A*) Sagittal 3D PD.(*B*) Coronal PD MPR of *A*. (*C*) Axial PD MPR. (*D*) Sagittal STIR.(*E*): Coronal T2 + FS.(*F*) Axial T2 + FS. FS, fat suppression; MPR, multiplanar reconstruction (of 3D scan); PD, proton density; STIR, short tau inversion recovery (sequence adequate for bone marrow edema evaluation).

little differences were found with regard to accuracy in evaluating small cartilage defects in the knee joint.[30] One of these MRI techniques is coherent oscillatory state acquisition for manipulation of image contrast (**Figs. 5** and **6**).

T2, T2*, and T1 rho mapping are well-validated techniques that evaluate the collagen network, GAGs, and water content in cartilage. They can be performed on most MR systems with a field strength of 1.5 T and higher. T2 mapping is particularly useful in assessing cartilage repair tissue after procedures such as microfracture, osteochondral grafting, and matrix-assisted autologous transplantation. One advantage of T2 mapping is that it does not require the administration of contrast material. However, it has long acquisition times when using a multi-echo spin-echo sequence. Additionally, physical activity has been found to impact cartilage T2 values.[31]

dGEMRIC is a technique that assesses the GAG content in cartilage. It is well validated and the measurements indirectly correlate with GAG content. However, dGEMRIC requires the use of intravenous contrast material with a time delay before image acquisition. The dGEMRIC index can be influenced by various physiologic factors, including exercise and body mass index.[17]

Table 2
Conventional anatomic MRI techniques

Technique	Strengths	Weakness
T1-weighted[a]	• Anatomic detail • Bone marrow evaluation, particularly differentiating red marrow from other pathology	• Poor contrast between cartilage and fluid • Poor detection of soft tissue edema • Not as sensitive as STIR or T2 with fat saturation for marrow edema
T2-weighted ± fat suppression[a]	• Good contrast between cartilage and fluid • At 3 T, T2-weighting with fat saturation is good for evaluation of cartilage and better than PD for evaluation of marrow pathology	• Frequency-selective fat-suppression may be incomplete due to local field inhomogeneities • Bone marrow edema detection poor without fat saturation
PD ± fat suppression[a]	• Good contrast between articular cartilage and joint fluid • Good for evaluation of internal cartilage signal	• Poor detection of fluid and marrow pathology without fat saturation • Susceptible to magic angle effects • Frequency-selective fat-suppression may be incomplete due to local field inhomogeneities
STIR	• Good for marrow and soft tissue pathology • Produces uniform fat saturation with less susceptibility to magnetic field inhomogeneities	• Poor SNR and CNR • Poor evaluation of cartilage
GRE	• High spatial resolution • Fibrocartilage • Detection of loose bodies and hemorrhage	• Poor detection of marrow pathology • Metallic hardware artifacts due to susceptibility

Abbreviations: CNR, contrast-to-noise ratio; GRE, gradient recalled echo; PD, proton density; STIR, short tau inversion recovery; SNR, signal-to-noise ratio.
[a] ICRS-recommended MRI sequences for evaluation of cartilage repair.

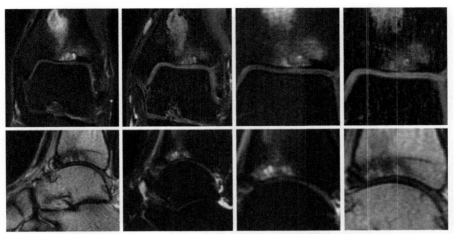

Fig. 5. MRI of a 45-year-old male 1 year after hyperdorsiflexion trauma. Osteochondral lesion in the distal tibia. Note cystic lesions of the subcortical bone limited cartilage damage. Right side shows close-up images. Note the added value of a novel 3D imaging technique and PD sequences compared to conventional, T1, and T2 images. Coronal images show PD (left) and 3D COSMIC right; sagittal images show T1 (left) and T2 (right) images. COSMIC, coherent oscillatory state acquisition for manipulation of image contrast; PD, proton density.

Diffusion-weighted imaging (DWI) evaluates the collagen network and GAGs in cartilage. It offers a short sequence duration and can differentiate between normal articular cartilage and repair tissue from procedures like microfracture and matrix-assisted autologous transplantation. DWI does not require the administration of contrast material. However, its semiquantitative image processing can be demanding, and it is susceptible to motion artifacts.[31]

MRI field strength

The field strength of the MRI scanner is an important consideration when imaging cartilage. Low-field scanners are generally limited in their ability to assess cartilage morphology and are not recommended for this purpose. However, recent advancements in image optimization through the use of artificial intelligence (AI) have shown promising results for imaging at low field strength, as low as 0.55 T. Imaging at this lower field strength with AI processing and optimization can yield similar sensitivity on cartilage pathologies compared to 1.5 T without a significant loss of diagnostic information.[32] These techniques can be advantageous, as low-field scanners offer shorter scanning protocols and reduce energy and helium consumption associated with powerful magnets. The current standard for imaging cartilage is 1.5 T, with most research conducted at this field strength. However, studies have demonstrated that 3.0 T MRI provides better visualization of cartilage lesions and may be more suitable for assessing focal cartilage abnormalities.[33,34] Cartilage volumetric measurements obtained at 3.0 T have been found to be more accurate than those obtained at 1.5 T. Additionally, 3.0 T MRI has shown superior ability to detect changes in cartilage status over time and evaluate responses to treatment with structure-modifying drugs. Thus, 3.0 T MRI has been deemed superior to 1.5 T MRI in visualizing cartilage lesions and assessing cartilage abnormalities.[33–35] MRI at 7.0 T is currently limited to research purposes. Available sequence protocols at 7.0 T have not demonstrated

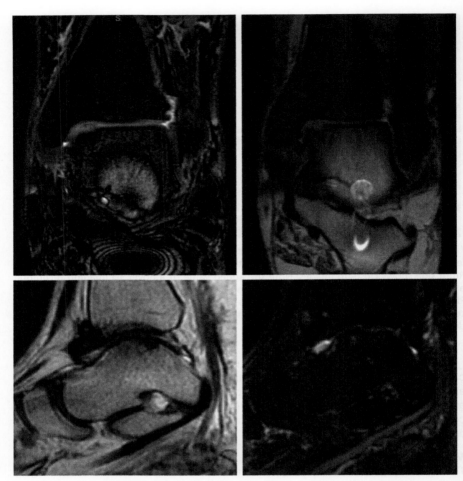

Fig. 6. MRI of a 50-year-old patient with OLT after repair with bone graft and BioCartilage repair. Left top: coronal COSMIC sequence, showing fibrocartilage layer visible as repair tissue and artifacts as a result of calcaneal screw placement after calcaneal osteotomy. Right top: coronal PD + FS. Left and right bottom: sagittal T1 and T2 images. COSMIC, coherent oscillatory state acquisition for manipulation of image contrast; FS, fat suppression; OLT, osteochondral lesion of the talus; PD, proton density.

superiority over 3.0 T for cartilage assessment.[36–38] Future research should focus on developing surface coils and optimized sequences specifically designed for 7.0 T imaging. Although image quality is similar at both 3.0 T and 7.0 T, challenges such as chemical shift artifacts and incomplete fat saturation have been observed at 7.0 T. Addressing these issues will further enhance the potential of 7.0 T MRI for cartilage imaging.

Scoring Systems of Cartilage

The classification of ankle osteochondral lesions, and its repair, has evolved over time with the introduction of new imaging modalities. In 1959, Berndt and Harty established the widely used 4-stage classification system based on the severity of the lesion seen on plain radiographs. This classification system continues to hold importance in evaluating plain radiographs.[39] With the use of CT, a fifth type was added based on CT findings, characterized by a radiolucent cystic lesion.[11] With the emergence of MRI as the gold standard imaging tool for diagnosing osteochondral lesions, several classifications based on MRI have been proposed, including an MRI-based classification for OLTs.[40] Subsequently, MRI was used to describe the condition of both the cartilage and subchondral bone, contributing to the understanding and characterization of osteochondral lesions.[41]

MRI Scoring Systems of Cartilage Repair

More recently, high-resolution MRI using microscopy coil imaging at 1.5 T or 3.0 T resulted in various scoring systems developed to assess the morphologic characteristics of cartilage repair after procedures.[42] The most commonly used system is MOCART (MR observation of cartilage repair tissue), which is a reproducible and semiquantitative scoring system (**Table 3**). It was developed by the ICRS to provide a comprehensive evaluation of the repaired tissue. MOCART evaluates 9 structural variables to assess imaging features related to cartilage repair.[43,44] MOCART is valuable for clinical follow-up and can be utilized to compare outcomes of different surgical techniques in longitudinal studies. Parameters such as defect fill and changes in subchondral bone show good correlation with clinical outcomes.[26] Another frequently used scoring system is the Henderson classification system, which considers factors like defect filling, cartilage signal intensity, subchondral edema, and joint effusion. This system provides insights into the degree of defect fill, cartilage condition, and presence of edema or effusion.[45] A meta-analysis study examined various MRI classification systems and features to determine their correlation with clinical outcomes following cartilage repair. The results revealed that the correlation between MRI findings and postsurgical outcomes varied depending on the type of surgery performed. For example, microfracture outcomes were strongly correlated with the MRI scores on subchondral edema and repair tissue signal. Autologous chondrocyte implantation

Table 3	
Magnetic Resonance Observation of Cartilage Repair Tissue Scoring system	
Degree of defect repair and defect filling	Complete: on a level with adjacent cartilage Hypertrophy: over the level of the adjacent cartilage Incomplete: under the level of the adjacent cartilage; underfilling
Integration to border zone	Complete: complete integration with adjacent cartilage Incomplete: incomplete integration with adjacent cartilage
Surface of the repair tissue	Surface intact: lamina intact Surface damaged: fibrillations, fissures and ulcerations
Structure of the repair tissue	Homogenous/Inhomogeneous or cleft formation
Signal intensity of the repair tissue	T2-weighted fast spin echo: isointense/mild hyperintense/marked hyperintense 3D gradient echo with fat suppression: isointense/mild hyperintense/marked hyperintense
Subchondral lamina	Intact/Not intact
Subchondral bone	Intact/Not intact: edema, granulation tissue, cysts, sclerosis
Adhesions	Yes/No
Effusion	Yes/No

outcomes showed significant correlation with regard to repair tissue signal and graft hypertrophy. OATS outcomes were most significantly correlated with osteochondral defect fill and repair tissue structure.[46] It is important to note that many MRI findings, such as hyperintense signal of repair tissue, subchondral edema, and effusion, may be part of the normal repair process. Therefore, MRI classification systems have limited utility in the early postoperative period. Overall, MRI scoring systems provide valuable information about cartilage repair morphology and can be helpful in assessing clinical outcomes. However, the specific correlations between MRI findings and surgical outcomes vary depending on the type of procedure performed.

Second-Look Arthroscopy

Second-look arthroscopy is a valuable procedure for directly visualizing repaired cartilage in order to assess the extent of healing, integration with surrounding tissue, and overall quality of the repair. It provides crucial information on factors such as defect filling, surface integrity, and stability of the repaired cartilage. The firmness of the cartilage can be evaluated using a probe, and visual inspection allows for assessment of color and smoothness.[25,47] Additionally, complications such as graft delamination, graft hypertrophy, fibrous tissue formation, or the presence of loose bodies can be identified. As such, there can be a mismatch between MRI findings and arthroscopy results. In approximately 24% of cases, MRI may lack details regarding cartilage firmness and integration into border zones.[26] Several scoring systems have been developed to arthroscopically assess repaired cartilage. Both the ICRS Score and the Oswestry Arthroscopic Score are frequently used and have been validated to evaluate repair tissue quality.[48]

However, it is important to note that second-look arthroscopy is primarily focused on the morphologic evaluation of cartilage and does not provide information about the underlying bone. Considering the invasiveness, associated risks, and costs of second-look arthroscopy, it is not recommended as a routine evaluation procedure for cartilage repair. Instead, it should be reserved for specific cases where there are concerns or uncertainties that cannot be adequately addressed through noninvasive imaging techniques.

PATIENT-REPORTED OUTCOME MEASURES

To determine the effectiveness of treatment, it is essential to define optimal outcomes. Current consensus defines treatment success based on several factors, including the absence of pain, patient satisfaction, return to preinjury work and sports levels, and improvement in pretreatment PROMs.[49] PROMs such as the Foot and Ankle Outcome Score (FOAS), the American Orthopedic Foot and Ankle Society (AOFAS) Score, visual analog scales, and patient satisfaction measures are commonly employed to assess treatment success.

The FAOS is a patient-reported outcome measure specifically designed to assess foot and ankle-related functional limitations, pain, and quality of life. It is commonly used in clinical practice and research to evaluate the effectiveness of interventions and track changes in foot and ankle conditions over time. The FAOS questionnaire has been validated and demonstrated good reliability and responsiveness in ankle sprains, Achilles tendon disorders, osteoarthritis, and ankle fractures. There was a significant correlation between the FAOS scores and ICRS grades.[26]

The AOFAS Ankle-Hindfoot Score: The AOFAS score is a widely used questionnaire that assesses ankle function and pain. It includes questions on pain, walking ability, range of motion, alignment, and patient satisfaction.

DISCUSSION

This review presents an overview of the current status of preoperative imaging modalities for osteochondral defects of the ankle joint. Furthermore it focuses on the assessment of cartilage repair, including imaging, arthroscopy, and PROMs. As such, it summarizes radiological evaluation techniques for assessing the impact of cartilage repair.

In the preoperative phase, MRI has become an indispensable noninvasive method for assessing changes in articular cartilage and subchondral bone. When it comes to detecting cartilage damage, MRI outperforms CT in terms of sensitivity. However, combining CT, with contrast-enhanced or CT arthrographic examinations can enhance the accuracy, bringing it closer to that of MRI.[18] It's worth noting that in the presence of significant bone edema, MRI images may overestimate the size of osteochondral defects. Nevertheless, with bone edema suppressing sequence protocols, MRI can still provide reliable estimations for cystic bone lesions, as can be observed in **Fig. 4**.[50] Therefore, when individuals experience persistent ankle pain despite negative radiographic findings, MRI is the preferred imaging modality as it allows for evaluation of both intra-articular and extra-articular findings, such as ligament or tendon injuries. On the other hand, when an osteochondral lesion is identified on plain radiographs, CT can be the preferred choice for further assessment, providing precise details about the size and location of the defect to assist in preoperative planning.[51,52]

There is an added value of SPECT/CT in the preoperative setting, as the osteoblastic activity shown on SPECT/CT is thought to have a high correlation with the source of the symptoms of the patient. It can show the precise location of activity, especially in the setting of multiple lesions.[20,21]

Postoperative radiographs are recommended, especially if bone grafting or medial malleolar osteotomy was performed.[12] In cases where patients continue to experience symptoms after surgery, MRI may be necessary. MRI provides valuable information on tissue repair, defect filling percentage, and integration of the repair tissue with the subchondral bone (refer to **Tables 1** and **3**). It is important to note that unexpected findings on MRI, such as persistent bone marrow edema, can occur even in the absence of clinical symptoms. For instance, bone marrow edema is commonly observed in patients who undergo osteochondral transplantation due to surgical penetration of the cortex, resulting in a reactive finding.[53] Several studies have evaluated the presence of edema and found no correlation with clinical outcomes.[46,53,54] However, in symptomatic patients, edema, which is often associated with poor integration, tends to become more pronounced over time. Subchondral bone marrow edema has been linked to inferior clinical outcomes, with patients experiencing persistent or new edema showing significantly lower AOFAS scores compared to those without edema. The disappearance of bone marrow edema is associated with significantly better clinical outcomes. Notably, the intensity of edema appears to be more relevant than its depth.[54–56] Postoperative MRI assessment of edema can be valuable for monitoring the healing status of the lesion and guiding further decision-making. However, in patients who meet criteria for good outcomes and do not have any other indications for MRI or longer follow-up, postoperative MRI may not be necessary.

Routine second-look arthroscopy is not recommended considering the invasiveness, associated risks, and costs, although the direct visualization and palpation of cartilage repair tissue allows for better evaluation of the repaired tissue.[26] The additional value in subsequent treatment steps has not been proven.

Numerous studies have examined prognostic factors that have a negative impact on the clinical outcomes of ankle cartilage lesion treatment, with lesion size being the most frequently mentioned factor, particularly those involving BMS.[57] However, the measurement and reporting of lesion size have varied across studies, with different methods such as diameter, area, volume, or depth being used. Thus, while the importance of lesion size is logical, its significance remains to be firmly established.

Subchondral edema, characterized by the accumulation of fluid in the bone beneath the cartilage, remains a topic of uncertainty regarding its prognostic and therapeutic implications. Shimozono and colleagues[58] found that the presence of subchondral bone marrow edema at midterm follow-up after BMS for OLTs was associated with worse clinical outcomes. The degree of subchondral bone marrow edema was also found to be correlated with poorer clinical outcomes. However, at short-term follow-up, no significant differences in clinical outcomes were observed based on the presence or degree of bone marrow edema, and no correlation was found between clinical outcomes and the degree of edema.

Similarly, subchondral cysts, commonly observed in the surgical management of OLT cases, were found to occur at the graft-host interface, indicating potential graft failure. Although the presence of subchondral cysts or bone marrow edema does not appear to impact short-term clinical outcomes significantly, their long-term effects remain uncertain. Savage-Elliott and colleagues[59] reported that 65% of patients who underwent autologous osteochondral transplantation had evidence of cystic changes on MRI at a mean follow-up of 15 months, yet no impact on clinical outcomes was detected in the short term.

In conclusion, it is essential to acknowledge that the lack of high-quality clinical evidence in this field has necessitated alternative methods for developing best practice guidelines. Nevertheless, MRI has benefited from advancements in techniques, improved coils, and stronger magnetic fields, leading to better imaging of cartilage. As such, MRI has become a crucial noninvasive imaging tool for diagnosing osteochondral lesions of the ankle and imaging its repair, with high diagnostic accuracy.

CLINICS CARE POINTS

Pearls:

- In instances where MRI is impractical, substitute imaging modalities such as contrast-enhanced or CT arthrographic examinations prove to be viable alternatives.
- The incorporation of SPECT/CT in the preoperative phase offers additional diagnostic value, exhibiting a significant correlation with the etiology of the patient's symptoms.
- The assessment of postoperative edema via MRI serves as a valuable tool for monitoring the progression of lesion healing.

Pitfalls:

- Postoperative MRI is deemed unnecessary for patients meeting criteria indicative of favorable outcomes, in the absence of other indications or a need for extended follow-up.

DISCLOSURE

The authors report no relationships, conditions, or circumstances that present a potential conflict of interest.

REFERENCES

1. Elias I, Zoga AC, Morrison WB, et al. Osteochondral lesions of the talus: localization and morphologic data from 424 patients using a novel anatomical grid scheme. Foot Ankle Int 2007;28(2):154–61.
2. Orr JD, Dutton JR, Fowler JT. Anatomic location and morphology of symptomatic, operatively treated osteochondral lesions of the talus. Foot Ankle Int 2012;33:1051–7.
3. Riaz O, Boyce Cam N, Shenolikar A. An osteochondral lesion in the distal fibula: a case report. Foot Ankle Spec 2012;5(6):394–6.
4. Dahmen J, Lambers KTA, Reilingh ML, et al. No superior treatment for primary osteochondral defects of the talus. Knee Surg Sports Traumatol Arthrosc 2018;26(7):2142–57.
5. Becher C, Driessen A, Hess T, et al. Microfracture for chondral defects of the talus: maintenance of early results at midterm follow-up. Knee Surg Sports Traumatol Arthrosc 2010;18(5):656–63.
6. Polat G, Erşen A, Erdil ME, et al. Long-term results of microfracture in the treatment of talus osteochondral lesions. Knee Surg Sports Traumatol Arthrosc 2016 Apr;24(4):1299–303.
7. Guelfi M, DiGiovanni CW, Calder J, et al. Large variation in management of talar osteochondral lesions among foot and ankle surgeons: results from an international survey. Knee Surg Sports Traumatol Arthrosc 2021;29(5):1593–603.
8. Kennedy JG, Murawski CD. The treatment of osteochondral lesions of the talus with autologous osteochondral transplantation and bone marrow aspirate concentrate: surgical technique. Cartilage 2011;2(4):327–36.
9. Bruns J, Habermann C, Werner M. Osteochondral lesions of the talus: a review on talus osteochondral injuries. Including Osteochondritis Dissecans. Cartilage 2021;13(1_suppl):1380S–401S.
10. Gianakos AL, Yasui Y, Hannon CP, et al. Current management of talar osteochondral lesions. World J Orthop 2017;8(1):12–20.
11. Loomer R, Fisher C, Lloyd-Smith R, et al. Osteochondral lesions of the talus. Am J Sports Med 1993;21(1):13–9.
12. Tandogan RN, Kayaalp A, Taşer O, et al. Evaluation of osteochondral lesions of the talus: comparison of plain radiography and contrast-enhanced MR imaging. Acta Orthop Traumatol Turc 2004;38(1):27–32.
13. Zumstein V, Kraljević M, Conzen A, et al. Thickness distribution of the glenohumeral joint cartilage: a quantitative study using computed tomography. Surg Radiol Anat 2014;36(4):327–31.
14. Hirvasniemi J, Kulmala KA, Lammentausta E, et al. In vivo comparison of delayed gadolinium-enhanced MRI of cartilage and delayed quantitative CT arthrography in imaging of articular cartilage. Osteoarthritis Cartilage 2013;21(3):434–42.
15. Bansal PN, Joshi NS, Entezari V, et al. Contrast enhanced computed tomography can predict the glycosaminoglycan content and biomechanical properties of articular cartilage. Osteoarthritis Cartilage 2010 Feb;18(2):184–91.
16. Nelson BB, Mäkelä JTA, Lawson TB, et al. Cationic contrast-enhanced computed tomography distinguishes between reparative, degenerative, and healthy equine articular cartilage. J Orthop Res 2021;39(8):1647–57.
17. Tiderius CJ, Svensson J, Leander P, et al. dGEMRIC (delayed gadolinium-enhanced MRI of cartilage) indicates adaptive capacity of human knee cartilage. Magn Reson Med 2004;51(2):286–90.

18. Kim DY, Yoon JM, Park GY, et al. Computed tomography arthrography versus magnetic resonance imaging for diagnosis of osteochondral lesions of the talus. Arch Orthop Trauma Surg 2023;143(9):5631–9.

19. Power SP, Moloney F, Twomey M, et al. Computed tomography and patient risk: Facts, perceptions and uncertainties. World J Radiol 2016;8(12):902–15.

20. Seo Y, Kim S, Yoon HJ, et al. The diagnostic value of 99mTc-HDP SPECT/CT for assessing bone marrow edema in patients with osteochondral lesions of the talus. Clin Orthop Surg 2020;12(3):345–51.

21. Meftah M, Katchis SD, Scharf SC, et al. SPECT/CT in the management of osteochondral lesions of the talus. Foot Ankle Int 2011;32(3):233–8.

22. Tamam C, Tamam MO, Yildirim D, et al. Diagnostic value of single-photon emission computed tomography combined with computed tomography in relation to MRI on osteochondral lesions of the talus. Nucl Med Commun 2015;36(8):808–14.

23. Henkelmann R, Röther J, Lauenstein TC, et al. Value of single photon emission computed tomography in the diagnostics of osteochondral lesions of the talus. Orthopä 2006;35(11):1149–55.

24. Tis JE, Cobetto NE, Sedory SE, et al. Application of SPECT/CT imaging in the foot and ankle. Foot Ankle Clin 2017;22(3):461–75.

25. Choi YR, Kim BS, Kim YM, et al. Second-look arthroscopic and magnetic resonance analysis after internal fixation of osteochondral lesions of the talus. Sci Rep 2022;12(1):10833.

26. Yang HY, Lee KB. Arthroscopic microfracture for osteochondral lesions of the talus: second-look arthroscopic and magnetic resonance analysis of cartilage repair tissue outcomes. J Bone Joint Surg Am 2020;102(1):10–20.

27. Liu YW, Tran MD, Skalski MR, et al. MR imaging of cartilage repair surgery of the knee. Clin Imaging 2019;58:129–39.

28. Walter SS, Fritz B, Kijowski R, et al. 2D versus 3D MRI of osteoarthritis in clinical practice and research. Skeletal Radiol 2023;52(11):2211–24.

29. Fritz B, Fritz J, Sutter R. 3D MRI of the ankle: a concise state-of-the-art review. Semin Musculoskelet Radiol 2021;25(3):514–26.

30. Chen CA, Kijowski R, Shapiro LM, et al. Cartilage morphology at 3.0T: assessment of three-dimensional magnetic resonance imaging techniques. J Magn Reson Imaging 2010;32(1):173–83.

31. Nieminen MT, Casula V, Nissi MJ. Compositional MRI of articular cartilage - current status and the way forward. Osteoarthritis Cartilage 2022;30(5):633–5.

32. Lopez Schmidt I, Haag N, Shahzadi I, et al. Diagnostic image quality of a low-field (0.55T) knee MRI Protocol using deep learning image reconstruction compared with a standard (1.5T) knee MRI protocol. J Clin Med 2023;12(5):1916.

33. Mandell JC, Rhodes JA, Shah N, et al. Routine clinical knee MR reports: comparison of diagnostic performance at 1.5 T and 3.0 T for assessment of the articular cartilage. Skeletal Radiol 2017;46(11):1487–98.

34. Springer E, Bohndorf K, Juras V, et al. Comparison of routine knee magnetic resonance imaging at 3 T and 7 T. Invest Radiol 2017;52(1):42–54.

35. Cheng Q, Zhao FC. Comparison of 1.5- and 3.0-T magnetic resonance imaging for evaluating lesions of the knee: A systematic review and meta-analysis (PRISMA- compliant article). Medicine (Baltim) 2018;97(38):e12401.

36. Heiss R, Weber MA, Balbach E, et al. Clinical application of ultrahigh-field-strength wrist mri: a multireader 3-t and 7-t comparison study. Radiology 2023;307(2):e220753.

37. Trattnig S, Bogner W, Gruber S, et al. Clinical applications at ultrahigh field (7 T). Where does it make the difference? NMR Biomed 2016;29(9):1316–34.

38. Friebe B, Richter M, Penzlin S, et al. Assessment of low-grade meniscal and cartilage damage of the knee at 7 t: a comparison to 3 t imaging with arthroscopic correlation. Invest Radiol 2018;53(7):390–6.

39. Berndt AL, Harty M. Transchondral fractures (osteochondritis dissecans) of the talus. J Bone Joint Surg Am 1959;41-A:988–1020.

40. Dipaola JD, Nelson DW, Colville MR. Characterizing osteochondral lesions by magnetic resonance imaging. Arthroscopy 1991;7(1):101–4.

41. Taranow WS, Bisignani GA, Towers JD, et al. Retrograde drilling of osteochondral lesions of the medial talar dome. Foot Ankle Int 1999;20(8):474–80.

42. Griffith JF, Lau DT, Yeung DK, et al. High-resolution MR imaging of talar osteochondral lesions with new classification. Skeletal Radiol 2012;41(4):387–99.

43. Marlovits S, Singer P, Zeller P, et al. Magnetic resonance observation of cartilage repair tissue (MOCART) for the evaluation of autologous chondrocyte transplantation: determination of interobserver variability and correlation to clinical outcome after 2 years. Eur J Radiol 2006;57(1):16–23.

44. Marlovits S, Striessnig G, Resinger CT, et al. Definition of pertinent parameters for the evaluation of articular cartilage repair tissue with high-resolution magnetic resonance imaging. Eur J Radiol 2004;52(3):310–9.

45. Henderson IJ, Tuy B, Connell D, et al. Prospective clinical study of autologous chondrocyte implantation and correlation with MRI at three and 12 months. J Bone Joint Surg Br 2003;85(7):1060–6.

46. Blackman AJ, Smith MV, Flanigan DC, et al. Correlation between magnetic resonance imaging and clinical outcomes after cartilage repair surgery in the knee: a systematic review and meta-analysis. Am J Sports Med 2013;41(6):1426–34.

47. Chun KC, Kim KM, Jeong KJ, et al. Arthroscopic bioabsorbable screw fixation of unstable osteochondritis dissecans in adolescents: clinical results, magnetic resonance imaging, and second-look arthroscopic findings. Clin Orthop Surg 2016;8(1):57–64.

48. Paatela T, Vasara A, Nurmi H, et al. Assessment of cartilage repair quality with the international cartilage repair society score and the oswestry arthroscopy score. J Orthop Res 2020;38(3):555–62.

49. van Dijk PAD, Murawski CD, Hunt KJ, et al, International Consensus Group on Cartilage Repair of the Ankle. International Consensus Group on Cartilage Repair of the Ankle. Post-treatment Follow-up, Imaging, and Outcome Scores: Proceedings of the International Consensus Meeting on Cartilage Repair of the Ankle. Foot Ankle Int 2018;39(1_suppl):68S–73S.

50. Deng E, Gao L, Shi W, et al. Both magnetic resonance imaging and computed tomography are reliable and valid in evaluating cystic osteochondral lesions of the talus. Orthop J Sports Med 2020;8(9). 2325967120946697.

51. Van Bergen CJ, Tuijthof GJ, Blankevoort L, et al. Computed tomography of the ankle in full plantar fexion: a reliable method for preoperative planning of arthroscopic access to osteochondral defects of the talus. Arthroscopy 2012;28: 985–992 37.

52. Van Bergen CJ, Tuijthof GJ, Maas M, et al. Arthroscopic accessibility of the talus quantifed by computed tomography simulation. Am J Sports Med 2012;40: 2318–24.

53. Link TM, Mischung J, Wörtler K, et al. Normal and pathological MR findings in osteochondral autografts with longitudinal follow-up. Eur Radiol 2006;16(1):88–96.

54. Marcacci M, Andriolo L, Kon E, et al. Bone marrow edema and results after cartilage repair. Ann Transl Med 2015;3(10):132.
55. Kuni B, Schmitt H, Chloridis D, et al. Clinical and MRI results after microfracture of osteochondral lesions of the talus. Arch Orthop Trauma Surg 2012;132(12): 1765–71.
56. Cuttica DJ, Shockley JA, Hyer CF, et al. Correlation of MRI edema and clinical outcomes following microfracture of osteochondral lesions of the talus. Foot Ankle Spec 2011;4(5):274–9.
57. Ramponi L, Yasui Y, Murawski CD, et al. Lesion size is a predictor of clinical outcomes after bone marrow stimulation for osteochondral lesions of the talus: a systematic review. Am J Sports Med 2017;45(7):1698–705.
58. Shimozono Y, Brown AJ, Batista JP, et al, International Consensus Group on Cartilage Repair of the Ankle. International consensus group on cartilage repair of the ankle. subchondral pathology: proceedings of the international consensus meeting on cartilage repair of the ankle. Foot Ankle Int 2018;39(1_suppl):48S–53S.
59. Savage-Elliott I, Smyth NA, Deyer TW, et al. Magnetic resonance imaging evidence of postoperative cyst formation does not appear to affect clinical outcomes after autologous osteochondral transplantation of the talus. Arthroscopy 2016;32(9):1846–54.

Conservative Treatment for Ankle Cartilage: Cellular and Acellular Therapies

A Systematic Review

Daniele Altomare, MD[a,b,*], Berardo Di Matteo, MD, PhD[a,b,c],
Elizaveta Kon, MD, PhD[a,b,c]

KEYWORDS

- Cartilage • Biological therapies • Ankle • Osteoarthritis
- Osteochondral lesion of talus • Conservative • Ankle injection

KEY POINTS

- A paucity of data are available about conservative biological therapies for ankle cartilage.
- The data available refer to small series with a bad methodological quality.
- Only one high methodological study is available, and it shows no beneficial effect over placebo for growth factors in ankle osteoarthritis.

INTRODUCTION

Ankle cartilage lesions and ankle osteoarthritis (OA) are high burden injuries for the patient, leading to a severe loss of quality of life and activity level.[1]

Despite the prevalence of cartilage lesion of the ankle is high, especially among young patients suffering ankle instability, ankle OA is not so frequent as for other joints, like knee or hip.

Ankle cartilage lesions, especially of the talus, were found to be present in almost a third of the patients with chronic lateral instability, which is a very common condition among population.[2,3]

As a matter of fact, ankle OA occurs as post-traumatic in most of cases (80%), in the context of rheumatoid disease in the 10% to 15% of cases, and it is idiopathic in just the remainder 5% to 10%.[4]

[a] Department of Biomedical Sciences, Humanitas University, Via Rita Levi Montalcini 4, Pieve Emanuele, Milan 20090, Italy; [b] Department of Orthopaedics and Traumatology, IRCCS Humanitas Research Hospital, Via Manzoni 56, Rozzano, Milan 20089, Italy; [c] Department of Traumatology, Orthopaedics and Disaster Surgery, Sechenov University, Moscow, 119991, Russia
* Corresponding author. Humanitas Clinical and Research Institute, Via A. Manzoni 113, Rozzano, Milan 20089, Italy.
E-mail address: dott.danielealtomare@gmail.com

Foot Ankle Clin N Am 29 (2024) 253–263
https://doi.org/10.1016/j.fcl.2023.07.003
1083-7515/24/© 2023 Elsevier Inc. All rights reserved.

Furthermore, giving the post-traumatic origin of ankle cartilage disease, both isolated lesion of cartilage and osteoarthritic degeneration, a high incidence of axial deformity is associated.[5]

Thus, the malalignment resulting in a mechanical overload of the joint contraindicates any conservative approach, both surgical (ie, bone marrow stimulation) or nonsurgical (intra-articular injection).

Clinical data about the efficiency of biological treatment in orthopedic are roughly rising among the literature. Despite the evidence of a proper regenerative role on the articular cartilage is lacking, many papers have described the potential beneficial role on joint homeostasis of injective therapies both cellular (ie, mesenchymal stem cells [MSCs]) and acellular (ie, platelet rich plasma [PRP]).[6–9]

Biological agents have been roughly investigated in other joint, especially in the knee, in the past few years. Despite the methodological quality of the studies is overall low, the constant increasing of data allowed to meta-analyze the literature, and Migliorini and colleagues[10] demonstrated promising clinical outcomes among randomized controlled trials (RCTs) for PRP. Nonetheless, the rising enthusiasm surrounding these new therapies could be misleading, and a high risk of publication bias should be recognized.

Given the smaller prevalence of ankle OA, and the relatively more severe degeneration of the joint of the affected patients, leading often to a surgical intervention, literature about the efficiency of biological treatments on the ankle is consistently lacking. Thus, especially in the ankle joint, there is a consistent lack of conservative therapeutic option for patients with cartilage disease.

The purpose of this review is to systematically analyze the current literature to retrieve any of the papers talking about biological acellular and cellular therapies for ankle cartilage disease, to better understand the potential therapeutic options available and the quality of the papers available.

The clinical relevance of the present study lies in letting the orthopedic surgeon educated about the current evidence of the new biological therapies for patients suffering of ankle cartilage disease.

Materials and Methods

A systematic review was performed on the literature about conservative injective treatment for ankle cartilage.

A search on PubMed, Medline, CINAHL, Cochrane, Embase, and Google Scholar databases was performed in April,2023 by the authors, using the following parameters: ("conservative treatment"[MeSH Terms] OR ("conservative"[All Fields] AND "treatment"[All Fields]) OR "conservative treatment"[All Fields]) AND ("cartilage"[MeSH Terms] OR "cartilage"[All Fields]) AND ("ankle"[MeSH Terms] OR "ankle"[All Fields] OR "ankle joint"[MeSH Terms] OR ("ankle"[All Fields] AND "joint"[All Fields]) OR "ankle joint"[All Fields]).

The PRISMA guidelines[11] (Preferred Reporting Items for Systematic Reviews and Meta-Analysis) were used to write the present review. A flowchart of the studies selection is presented in **Fig. 1**.

Firstly, title and abstract were screened. Inclusion criteria were as follows: (1) clinical reports of any level of evidence, (2) written in the English language, (3) published from 2013 to 2023, and (4) dealing with the nonsurgical use of cellular or acellular infiltrative therapies for ankle cartilage. All surgery-related articles, duplicate articles, articles from non-peer reviewed journals or articles lacking access to the full text, paper about animal models, conference presentations, narrative reviews, editorials, and expert opinions were excluded.

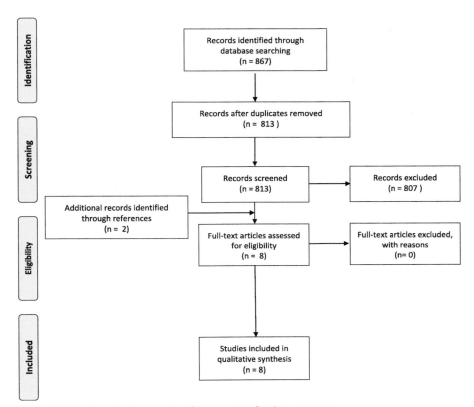

Fig. 1. PRIMA flowchart resuming the papers' selection process.

In second, full texts of selected articles were obtained and screened.

Reference lists from the selected papers were also screened, and 2 additional papers were included.

Eventually, 8 studies were included in the systematic review.

The study screening and selection were performed separately by 2 independent authors (B.D.M) and (D.A). Discrepancies between the 2 reviewers were resolved by discussion and consensus, and the final results were reviewed by the senior investigators. All the data retrieved from the analysis of the studies included in the present review have been summarized in **Table 1**.

Relevant data were collected in a Microsoft Excel 2017 sheet.

Given the heterogeneity of the data collected, it was not possible to pool them and perform a meta-analysis. Therefore, no statistical tests have been used. A descriptive analysis and qualitative synthesis of data were provided in the present systematic review.

Given the nature of the present paper (systematic review of the literature), no ethical approval was required.

RESULTS

Eight papers, published between 2013 and 2023, were finally included in the present review.

Summary of the included studies is presented in **Table 1**.

Table 1
Synopsis of the included studies

Author	Type of Study	Injected Product	Patients (n, M/F), Age, Symptoms	Follow-up	Main Findings
Paget et al,[12] 2021	Randomized double-blind placebo-controlled trial	*PRP* Arthrex ACP double Syringe System (Arthrex, Naples, FL) *Saline solution*	48 (26M; 22F), 54.8 ± 13.3 5 mo 52 (29M; 23F), 56.4 ± 14.4) 8 mo	26 mo	Among patients with ankle OA, PRP injections did not improve ankle symptoms over placebo.
Sun et al,[13] 2021	Prospective cohort	*PRP:* PLUS platelet concentrate separator (TCM biotech International Corp., Taiwan)	39 (22M; 17F), 55.5 ± 8.8 y of age 31 mo	6 mo	Significative reduction of symptoms at various scores over the course of 6 mo after the procedure in patients with ankle OA. The study support safety and effectiveness of single PRP injection for 6 mo.
Akpancar & Gul,[14] 2019	Retrospective comparative	*PRP:* GPS III platelet Separation System (Biomet Biologics) *Prolotherapy:* 2 mL 25% dextrose plus lidocaine	22 (6M; 12F) 54.0 ± 11.5 23.1 ± 22.4 mo 27 (8M; 19F, 57.7 ±11.1 y of age); 26.2 ± 16.8 mo	12 mo 12 mo	Improvement in pain and ankle function for both treatment at 1 y of follow-up for osteochondal lesions of talus.
Repetto et al,[15] 2017	Retrospective cohort	*PRP:* 3x Centrifugations of 450 mL blood sample	20 (12M; 8F; 57.5 y, 26 mean mo before injection)	17,7 +- 6,5 mo	PRP injection is a safe and effective option to postpone surgery in patients with ankle OA.
Fukawa et al,[16] 2017	Prospective cohort	*PRP:* Blood Separation Pack (Kawasumi Ltd.)	20 (5M; 15F; 59.3 ± 11.4 y of age)	6 mo	Single shot of intra-articular PRP significantly reduced pain in the patients with ankle OA.

Study	Study design	Intervention	n (age)	Follow-up	Outcomes
Emadedin et al,[18] 2015	Prospective cohort	MSCs: harvested from iliac crest, expanded in vitro and then injected	6	30 mo	Improvements in visual analogue score (VAS), Western Ontario and McMaaster University (WOMAC) Osteoarthritis index score, walking distance without pain in patients with ankle OA.
Angthong et al,[17] 2013	Retrospective cohort	PRP: Arthrex ACP double Syringe System (Arthrex, Naples, FL)	5 (50.8 ± 14.3)	13.88–18.38 mo	Post-treatment VAS score and short form health survey 36 (SF-36) were significantly higher than the mean pretreatment VAS score.
Hauser & Orlofsky,[19] 2013	Case report (1 ankle OA in a case series of 7 patients)	Tibial bone marrow: EZ-IO intraosseous access system	1 (F, 3 y duration of symptoms)	8 mo	Walking distance without pain improved in the patient from 30 ft to 2 miles after the treatment.

Acellular Therapies

Paget and colleagues[12] published the results of the first ever RCTs available on the literature about PRP injection in ankle OA. Over a mean follow-up of 26 months, PRP showed no beneficial effects over placebo.

Sun and colleagues[13] reported encouraging results for a single shot injection of PRP in a cohort of patients with ankle OA, obtaining a partial relief of symptoms at 6 months.

Akpancar and Gül[14] compared PRP injections to prolotherapy in patients with ostheocondral lesions of talus, reporting good clinical results for both therapies.

Repetto and colleagues[15] reported an original article about the results about the usage of PRP in a cohort of patients with high graded ankle OA and surgical indication for ankle fusion. PRP was effective in postpone surgery, giving a partial relief of symptoms.

Fukawa and colleagues[16] prospectively analyzed the effects of a single-shot injection of PRP in patients with ankle OA. Despite a short follow-up of 6 months, the treatment decreased significatively pain scores in the included patients.

Angthong and colleagues[17] reported relief of pain and improved quality of life in 5 patients affected by ankle OA, treated with a cycle of PRP injection.

Cellular Therapies

Emadedin and colleagues[18] harvested MSCs from the iliac crest of 6 patients with ankle OA. They subsequently injected in the ankle after in vitro expansion, reporting good clinical results at 30 months of follow-up.

Hauser and colleagues[19] reported a case series of 7 patients with OA treated with injection of tibial bone marrow. One of the included patients was affected by ankle OA: this patient had a beneficial effect from the procedure improving his walking distance without pain from 30 feet to 2 miles.

DISCUSSION

The main findings of the present review are as follows: (i) there is paucity of study available in literature about the conservative infiltrative therapies for ankle cartilage disease, (ii) the few available studies except one[12] showed a poor methodological quality, (iii) the only RCT available[12] showed no superiority of PRP over placebo. Given the present findings, although a big hope is placed in biological therapies for cartilage disease, this review showed that these therapies could not be recommended at the moment to address cartilage disease in tibiotarsal joint. Furthermore, given the paucity of papers available, a possible publication bias should be considered: authors approaching prospectively patients with this new group of therapies could be discouraged to publish about poor results, and on the other hand indexed journals could be discouraged to accept paper with a bad study design and reporting poor outcomes.

Interest about biological therapies (also known as: "Orthobiologics") in knee and hip OA has been rising consistently over the course of the last few decades. Despite many papers are showing encouraging results, and a certain beneficial effect especially on restoring joint homeostasis[20] could be recognized, clinical results are still controversial and the available meta-analysis show no superiority over control cohorts.[21]

Ankle OA is way less frequent than hip OA and knee OA, and way more often secondary to trauma or other medical conditions (ie, rheumatic arthritis), rather than idiopathic.[22] Given the etiology, patients suffering ankle OA often refer to the clinicians at a higher stage of OA, rather than mild OA. As a matter of fact, in most of the here included papers ankle OA gradation is reported: in most cases patients have high degrees of ankle OA. Repetto and colleagues[15] included patients with advanced OA which already received a surgical indication for ankle fusion; in the series by Fukawa and colleagues[16] the 65% of patients are Tanaka grade 3b or 4; in the RCT by Paget and colleagues[12] patients included are at least Kellgren-Lawrence II and two-third of the population included is grade 3 and 4. Addressing this kind of joint degeneration with conservative therapies should not lead to great expectations from a clinical point of view: a high risk of placebo effect should be expected and the paper by Paget[12] confirms the expectations. Furthermore, ankle OA is a disease with very changing symptoms: could be reasonable to think that the patients included in prospective cohorts referred to the orthopedic once in an active phase of their disease. Thus, the partial good results reported by the small series included could be misleading. In this scenario, the study by Paget[12] adds important elements to better contextualize the results reported by the other papers available. This scenario is superimposable to the knee one, in which a multiple of studies reported promising results for biological therapies but showing no superiority over the conventional treatments like hyaluronic acid (HA) injections.[23] The placebo effects of the intraarticular injection has been widely described, especially in OA.[24] The safety reported by the greatest part of the paper reporting results of intra-articular ankle injection[25] could let the orthopedic to give a try to the treatment. Nonetheless, the poor results of the reported papers cannot allow to define intra-articular ankle injection recommendable, especially talking about biological agents.

Acellular therapies include growth factors like PRP. PRP has becoming more and more popular and widely available over the course of the past decades. Even if their "regenerative" potential has been widely resized lately, growth factors like PRP could have a restoring effect on the joint homeostasis. In the present series of papers, the majority focused on the role of growth factors (PRP). Akpancar and colleagues[14] is the only one to combine a therapeutic arm with prolotherapy that consists in an injection of an irritative solution in the joint and that will not be discussed as a biological agent. However, in many countries prolotherapy is considered same as a placebo, and considering the superimposable results to PRP group, these results could further corroborate the thesis of Paget and colleagues.[12] Sun and colleagues[13] and Fukawa and colleagues[16] treated patients affected by ankle OA with a cycle and a single shot of PRP, respectively. In both studies the follow-up evaluation was at 6 months, and both reported good results especially in terms of pain. These papers, in the opinion of the senior authors, cannot provide any valid information to the current knowledge because the results cannot be divided by the natural course of the symptoms of OA, so a high risk of placebo effect should be considered for this short follow-up. On the other hand, both studies could provide strong evidence about the safety of the procedure, with a very risible number of complications detected. As a further factor of confusion, of the 6 papers including PRP therapy, only 2[12,17] used the same system (Arthrex ACP double Syringe System; Arthrex, Naples, FL).

Repetto and colleagues[15] treated with PRP patients with severe OA and a surgical indication to evaluate if PRP could postpone surgery of ankle fusion, maintaining a good quality of life and controlling symptoms. This strategy is interesting because can better highlight the role on joint homeostasis of growth factors.[6] In the opinion of the senior author, especially if considering a highly loaded joint like ankle, growth factors (GFs) alone can barely restore a good layer of cartilage, but can otherwise address the synovial tissue to better control inflammation and thus symptoms. The study by Repetto and colleagues[15] demonstrated this possible beneficial effect even in joints at "the end" of their degeneration path.

Cellular therapies, including MSCs harvested from adipose tissue and/or bone marrow, showed good results in knee OA[23] even though remaining nonsuperior to conventional treatments like hyaluronic acid (HA) injections. Talking about cellular therapies for ankle OA, literature is almost empty at the moment. In fact, the need for an anesthesia to harvest (ie, from iliac crest or tibial tuberosity) led the literature to be richer in papers in which the injection of MSCs was associated to surgery.[26]

Results are overall good, but once more the quality of the literature available is very low.[27–29]

A systematic review by Seow and colleagues[26] analyzed the available literature about augmentation with orthobiologics to bone marrow stimulation in osteochondral lesion of the talus. Despite a good number of papers retrieved, the evidence provided was limited, and no augmentation of bone marrow stimulation techniques (ie, micro-fractures) showed better results than augmentation with placebo or HA. The systematic review confirms that the use of cellular biological agents is preferred as an augmentation of surgery and not as a conservative therapy alone. Especially referring to isolated ostheochondral lesions of the talus the paucity of literature available could be referred to the preferable choice of a surgical option for this kind of lesion, given the good results for surgery reported in literature, even if considered biologically augmented (ie, autologous matrix-induced chondrogenesis procedure). Standing the current literature, bone marrow stimulation ± biological augmentation is a viable solution to treat osteochondral lesion of talus both in terms of safety and clinical results.[26] In the present scenario, a conservative approach to these patients, even if powered by biological agents, should not be indicated. In the here included papers, only 6 patients overall were treated by cellular therapies (5 in the series by Emadedin and colleagues[18] and 1 in the series of Hauser and colleagues[19]). In the opinion of the senior author, given the load of the ankle joint, the expectations on the potential beneficial effect of cellular therapies to restore a working layer of cartilage in single larger defect of cartilage or even more in a osteochondral lesion are too high, and thus these therapies should remain associated with operative procedures.

Although injective therapies, including HA, for ankle cartilage is not recommended routinely by International Orthopedics societies, evidence in literature over the past 2 decades has showed a certain beneficial effect: Boffa and colleagues[23] systematically analyzed the available literature to evaluate evidence supporting safety and effectiveness of injective treatment in osteochondral lesions of the talus and ankle OA, reporting safety and low relative efficacy versus placebo for HA injections. Evidence about other conservative approaches for ankle OA and Osteochondral lesion of Talus (OLT) in literature are poor but must be mentioned. A Cochrane Database Systematic review by Witteveen and colleagues[30] highlighted the absence of any RCTs for other conservative treatment out of HA injections for ankle OA. Papers about physical therapies and rehabilitation are lacking. Markovic and colleagues[31] systematically analyzed the literature about pulsed electromagnetic field therapy in osteoarthritis: they included 69 studies, of which only 1[32] included outcomes in ankle OA.

Limitations of the present paper are few and must be mentioned. First, the greater limitation in the opinion of the authors is derived by the limited number of papers available in literature. Overall, literature about conservative approach in ankle cartilage disease is very poor. Thus, the clinical of the present review is limited and this makes very difficult to give a day-by-day guideline of approach for the management of the patient. Second, the poor quality of the included papers, and the heterogeneity of the reported results did not allow a meta-analysis.

In conclusion, this review highlights the severe lack of literature about conservative therapies for ankle OA and OLT, especially regarding biological therapies. Given the current literature, biological therapies seem to be not recommendable to address ankle cartilage pathologies. Nonetheless, given the unexplored horizon of the potential of biological therapies and the ever-increasing number of patients suffering from ankle pathologies, it is mandatory to enlarge the field of clinical research about this topic.

CLINICS CARE POINTS

- Current evidence upon literature is insufficient to recommend conservative approach to ankle cartilage disease with cellular or acellular "orthobiologics" therapies.
- "Orthobiologics" in ankle cartilage disease could be beneficial as augmentation to surgery.
- Publication bias risk on this specific field is very high due the paucity of literature available and due the encouraging results of the application of these therapies in other joints, like knee.
- The slightly good results described by prospective cohort and retrospective cohort could be linked to a high risk of placebo effect.
- In the opinion of the senior author, use of *orthobiologics* in ankle cartilage disease should be limited to selected patients.

CONFLICT OF INTEREST STATEMENT

No conflict of interest to declare.

FUNDING SOURCE STATEMENT

This research did not receive any specific grant from funding agencies in the public, commercial, or not-for-profit sectors.

CONSENT TO PUBLISHING

All the authors have read and approved the content of the present article, which has not been submitted or published elsewhere. All the authors give their approval to the publication of the present paper in case of acceptance.

ETHICS STATEMENT

Given the nature of the present paper (systematic review of the literature), no ethical approval is required.

REFERENCES

1. Kolar M, Brulc U, Stražar K, et al. Patient-reported joint status and quality of life in sports-related ankle disorders and osteoarthritis. Int Orthop 2021;45(4):1049–55.
2. Wijnhoud EJ, Rikken QGH, Dahmen J, et al. One in Three Patients With Chronic Lateral Ankle Instability Has a Cartilage Lesion [published online ahead of print, 2022 Apr 6]. Am J Sports Med 2022. https://doi.org/10.1177/03635465221084365. 3635465221084365.
3. Michels F, Wastyn H, Pottel H, et al. The presence of persistent symptoms 12 months following a first lateral ankle sprain: A systematic review and meta-analysis. Foot Ankle Surg 2022;28(7):817–26.
4. Saltzman CL, Salamon ML, Blanchard GM, et al. Epidemiology of ankle arthritis: report of a consecutive series of 639 patients from a tertiary orthopaedic center. Iowa Orthop J 2005;25:44–6.

5. Maccario C, Paoli T, Romano F, et al. Transfibular total ankle arthroplasty : a new reliable procedure at five-year follow-up. Bone Joint J 2022;104-B(4):472–8.

6. Kim JG, Rim YA, Ju JH. The Role of Transforming Growth Factor Beta in Joint Homeostasis and Cartilage Regeneration. Tissue Eng Part C Methods 2022;28(10):570–87.

7. Lopa S, Colombini A, Moretti M, et al. Injective mesenchymal stem cell-based treatments for knee osteoarthritis: from mechanisms of action to current clinical evidences. Knee Surg Sports Traumatol Arthrosc 2019;27(6):2003–20.

8. Fusco G, Gambaro FM, Di Matteo B, et al. Injections in the osteoarthritic knee: a review of current treatment options. EFORT Open Rev 2021;6(6):501–9.

9. Szwedowski D, Szczepanek J, Paczesny Ł, et al. The Effect of Platelet-Rich Plasma on the Intra-Articular Microenvironment in Knee Osteoarthritis. Int J Mol Sci 2021;22(11):5492.

10. Filardo G, Previtali D, Napoli F, et al. PRP Injections for the Treatment of Knee Osteoarthritis: A Meta-Analysis of Randomized Controlled Trials. Cartilage 2021; 13(1_suppl):364S–75S.

11. Page MJ, McKenzie JE, Bossuyt PM, et al. The PRISMA 2020 statement: an updated guideline for reporting systematic reviews. BMJ 2021;372:n71.

12. Paget LDA, Reurink G, de Vos RJ, et al. Effect of Platelet-Rich Plasma Injections vs Placebo on Ankle Symptoms and Function in Patients With Ankle Osteoarthritis: A Randomized Clinical Trial. JAMA 2021;326(16):1595–605.

13. Sun SF, Hsu CW, Lin GC, et al. Efficacy and Safety of a Single Intra-articular Injection of Platelet-rich Plasma on Pain and Physical Function in Patients With Ankle Osteoarthritis-A Prospective Study. J Foot Ankle Surg 2021;60(4):676–82.

14. Akpancar S, Gül D. Comparison of Platelet Rich Plasma and Prolotherapy in the Management of Osteochondral Lesions of the Talus: A Retrospective Cohort Study. Med Sci Monit 2019;25:5640–7.

15. Repetto I, Biti B, Cerruti P, et al. Conservative Treatment of Ankle Osteoarthritis: Can Platelet-Rich Plasma Effectively Postpone Surgery? J Foot Ankle Surg 2017;56(2):362–5.

16. Fukawa T, Yamaguchi S, Akatsu Y, et al. Safety and Efficacy of Intra-articular Injection of Platelet-Rich Plasma in Patients With Ankle Osteoarthritis. Foot Ankle Int 2017;38(6):596–604.

17. Angthong C, Khadsongkram A, Angthong W. Outcomes and quality of life after platelet-rich plasma therapy in patients with recalcitrant hindfoot and ankle diseases: a preliminary report of 12 patients. J Foot Ankle Surg 2013;52(4):475–80.

18. Emadedin M, Ghorbani Liastani M, Fazeli R, et al. Long-Term Follow-up of Intra-articular Injection of Autologous Mesenchymal Stem Cells in Patients with Knee, Ankle, or Hip Osteoarthritis. Arch Iran Med 2015;18(6):336–44.

19. Hauser RA, Orlofsky A. Regenerative injection therapy with whole bone marrow aspirate for degenerative joint disease: a case series. Clin Med Insights Arthritis Musculoskelet Disord 2013;6:65–72.

20. Kon E, Di Matteo B, Delgado D, et al. Platelet-rich plasma for the treatment of knee osteoarthritis: an expert opinion and proposal for a novel classification and coding system. Expert Opin Biol Ther 2020;20(12):1447–60.

21. Delanois RE, Sax OC, Chen Z, et al. Biologic Therapies for the Treatment of Knee Osteoarthritis: An Updated Systematic Review. J Arthroplasty 2022;37(12):2480–506.

22. Valderrabano V, Horisberger M, Russell I, et al. Etiology of ankle osteoarthritis. Clin Orthop Relat Res 2009;467(7):1800–6.

23. Boffa A, Di Martino A, Andriolo L, et al. Bone marrow aspirate concentrate injections provide similar results versus viscosupplementation up to 24 months of follow-up in patients with symptomatic knee osteoarthritis. A randomized controlled trial. Knee Surg Sports Traumatol Arthrosc 2022;30(12):3958–67.
24. Bennell KL, Paterson KL, Metcalf BR, et al. Effect of Intra-articular Platelet-Rich Plasma vs Placebo Injection on Pain and Medial Tibial Cartilage Volume in Patients With Knee Osteoarthritis: The RESTORE Randomized Clinical Trial. JAMA 2021;326(20):2021–30.
25. Boffa A, Previtali D, Di Laura Frattura G, et al. Evidence on ankle injections for osteochondral lesions and osteoarthritis: a systematic review and meta-analysis. Int Orthop 2021;45(2):509–23.
26. Seow D, Ubillus HA, Azam MT, et al. Limited evidence of adjuvant biologics with bone marrow stimulation for the treatment of osteochondral lesion of the talus: a systematic review. Knee Surg Sports Traumatol Arthrosc 2022;30(12):4238–49.
27. Glenn R, Johns W, Walley K, et al. Topical Review: Bone Marrow Aspirate Concentrate and Its Clinical Use in Foot and Ankle Surgery. Foot Ankle Int 2021;42(9):1205–11.
28. Murphy EP, Fenelon C, McGoldrick NP, et al. Bone Marrow Aspirate Concentrate and Microfracture Technique for Talar Osteochondral Lesions of the Ankle. Arthrosc Tech 2018;7(4):e391–6.
29. Chahla J, Cinque ME, Shon JM, et al. Bone marrow aspirate concentrate for the treatment of osteochondral lesions of the talus: a systematic review of outcomes [published correction appears in J Exp Orthop. 2016. J Exp Orthop 2016;3(1):33.
30. Witteveen AG, Hofstad CJ, Kerkhoffs GM. Hyaluronic acid and other conservative treatment options for osteoarthritis of the ankle. Cochrane Database Syst Rev 2015;2015(10):CD010643.
31. Markovic L, Wagner B, Crevenna R. Effects of pulsed electromagnetic field therapy on outcomes associated with osteoarthritis : A systematic review of systematic reviews. Wien Klin Wochenschr 2022;134(11–12):425–33.
32. Trock DH, Bollet AJ, Dyer RH Jr, et al. A double-blind trial of the clinical effects of pulsed electromagnetic fields in osteoarthritis. J Rheumatol 1993;20(3):456–60.

Fixation of Osteochondral Lesions of the Talus

Indications, Techniques, Outcomes, and Pearls from the Amsterdam Perspective

Quinten G.H. Rikken, BSc[a,b,c],
Gino M.M.J. Kerkhoffs, MD, PhD[a,b,c],*

KEYWORDS

• OLT • Cartilage • Ankle • Talus • Fixation

KEY POINTS

- Symptomatic acute or chronic fragmentous osteochondral lesion of the talus (OLT) should always be considered for in situ fixation.
- Pre-treatment imaging, by means of computed tomography scanning or MR imaging, is helpful in clinical decision-making.
- Lesion and patient characteristics guide the treatment algorithm for fixation of fragmentous OLT.
- Choice of type and number of screws, or alternative fixation methods, is based on lesion and fragment morphology, size, and thickness, and should ideally be with 2 screws or pins or pegs in order to provide axial and rotational stability.
- Fixation of OLT can be through an arthroscopic or open approach and yields good clinical outcomes with union rates ranging from 77% to 100%.
- If fixation fails and/or results in a symptomatic non-union or malunion, all other surgical cartilage treatments for OLT are still feasible.

INTRODUCTION

The treatment of osteochondral lesions of the talus (OLT) remains a topic of debate as no superior treatment for primary or non-primary (ie, failed prior surgical treatment) lesions has yet been identified.[1,2] The current consensus is that it is crucial to incorporate

[a] Department of Orthopedic Surgery and Sports Medicine, Amsterdam Movement Sciences, Amsterdam UMC, Location AMC, University of Amsterdam, Meibergdreef 9, Amsterdam 1105 AZ, the Netherlands; [b] Academic Center for Evidence Based Sports Medicine (ACES), Amsterdam UMC, Amsterdam, the Netherlands; [c] Amsterdam Collaboration for Health and Safety in Sports (ACHSS), International Olympic Committee (IOC) Research Center, Amsterdam UMC, Amsterdam, the Netherlands
* Corresponding author.
E-mail address: g.m.kerkhoffs@amsterdamumc.nl

Foot Ankle Clin N Am 29 (2024) 265–279
https://doi.org/10.1016/j.fcl.2023.07.004
1083-7515/24/© 2023 Elsevier Inc. All rights reserved.

lesion and patient characteristics into the treatment algorithm for symptomatic OLT.[3-6] Herein, the identification of succinct morphologic lesion types, including crater morphology, the presence of a cyst, or fragment, has been an important topic of discussion as these may influence clinical outcomes as well as treatment choice.[3,4]

One such a morphologic lesion type is the fragmentous osteochondral lesion. These lesions may be amendable for, and can benefit from, in situ fixation.[4] The theoretic advantages of fixation over other surgical treatments for OLT are the retainment of the native hyaline cartilage, direct stabilization of the fragment, and high-quality subchondral bone repair.[7,8] To date, the procedure has shown promising outcomes with varying techniques, which makes it a valuable treatment option to consider by physicians who treat patients with OLT.[8-15] It is paramount that clinicians are up-to-date on the latest developments in this field. The goal of this current concepts review is therefore to describe the evidence-based clinical work-up, indications, surgical techniques, outcomes, and clinical pearls for fixation techniques of OLT from the Amsterdam perspective.

CLINICAL AND RADIOLOGICAL EVALUATION OF OSTEOCHONDRAL LESIONS OF THE TALUS
Clinical Evaluation and Initial Presentation

Up to 75% of patients with an OLT present after an ankle trauma, such as a sprain or fracture.[16,17] Patients with an osteochondral lesion typically present 6 to 12 months after initial injury with complaints of deep ankle pain during or after weight bearing.[3] Other complaints may be swelling, range of motion restriction, (pseudo) instability, or locking. The clinical evaluation comprises a thorough history and physical examination of the patient and their ankle complaints, including prior treatment, and is critical for establishing the correct treatment indication. Upon physical examination, physicians may observe a recognizable deep pain with direct palpation of the lesion or swelling.[3] Additionally, clinicians should assess the presence of concomitant injuries such as fractures, instability injuries, and impingement, as OLT frequently present alongside co-pathologies.[18-20] When a symptomatic OLT is suspected, additional imaging studies are indicated.

When considering the chronicity of the injury, one can separate distinct clinical presentations. In cases of a fragmentous osteochondral lesion, patients can present acutely after trauma (<6 weeks) with an osteochondral fracture (more likely to be located on the lateral talus–**Fig. 1**A) or as an acute on chronic lesion (rounded fragment with clearly demarcated sclerotic subchondral borders, suggesting a chronic component—as depicted in **Fig. 1**B), which may have already been present but can become symptomatic due to trauma.

In delayed or chronic (>6 weeks) lesions, these could present as a fragment with sub-fragmentous cysts (**Fig. 2**A) or as a crater with fragment remnants (ie, small fragment remaining in the original fragment bed—**Fig. 2**B). Another presentation is an asymptomatic lesion, which is most often encountered as an accidental finding on imaging studies, and may also present bilaterally.[21]

Radiological Evaluation

The first-line imaging tools for assessing a suspected OLT are computed tomography (CT)-scanning and MR-imaging as they both display a high diagnostic accuracy for OLT.[22] Additional weight-bearing radiographs can be obtained for assessing foot and ankle alignment and joint space narrowing when investigating degenerative changes of the joint. The authors prefer the utilization of CT for assessing the lesion and a

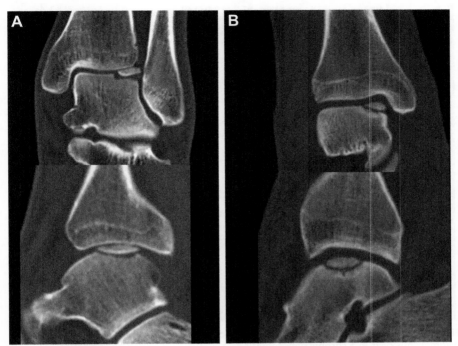

Fig. 1. (*A*) Depiction of an acute and displaced (inverted) symptomatic osteochondral fracture of the lateral talus in an 18-year- old elite-level ice skater after a pronation trauma. The patient is eligible for immediate fixation. (*B*) Osteochondral lesion with a rounded fragment in situ. Note the subchondral sclerotic changes and small cyst in the lesion bed. Such a lesion type may fit with an acute on chronic or asymptomatic presentation.

possible fragment as it allows for the detailed assessment of its bony morphology and size, which is crucial for treatment choice.[3,23] MR imaging is known to overestimate lesion size due to bone marrow edema, and in the experience of the authors may be less suited for assessing the bony morphology of the lesion and fragment.[24]

On imaging, the following aspects should be assessed: lesion size (coronal diameter, sagittal diameter, and depth), lesion morphology and the presence of a possible osteochondral fragment,[21] lesion location according to a 9-grid scheme,[25] possible coexisting tibial osteochondral lesions, degenerative changes,[26] and loose bodies. In case an osteochondral fragment is present, it is crucial to assess the following aspects: fragment dimensions (coronal diameter, sagittal diameter, and depth), fragment morphology, which may include the presence of possible sub-fragments cysts, interfragmentary fractures, and fragment stability (ie, displaced or non-displaced). Examples of different fragment morphologies are depicted in **Figs. 1–3**. Additional MR imaging can be obtained in case there is doubt about the integrity of the articular cartilage of the fragment, such as in non-primary lesions, or when necessary for the diagnosis of any co-pathology of the foot and ankle.

INDICATIONS FOR FIXATION

When considering a fixation procedure, it is important to consider lesion and patient factors in order to determine the eligibility as well as the optimal technique.[3,4]

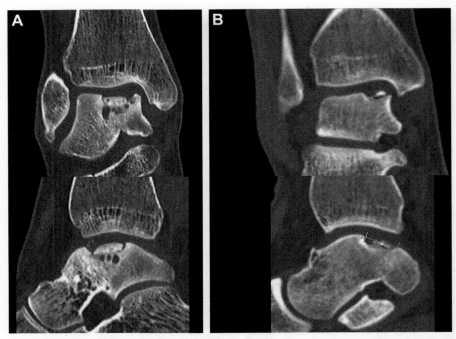

Fig. 2. Examples of different lesion types in chronic lesions. (*A*) Fragmentous OLT with sub-fragmentous cysts in a chronic symptomatic case, which underwent open fixation with sub-chondral filling with autologous bone. Note the extensive sub-fragmentous cyst formation, suggestive of a chronic process and/or instable fragment. (*B*) Medial OLT with crater morphology and a small fragment remnant in situ.

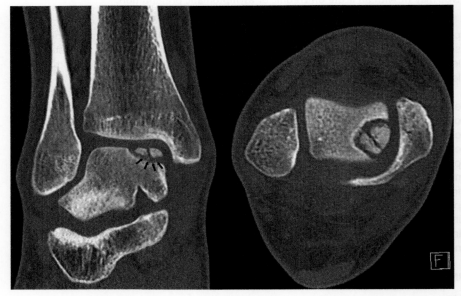

Fig. 3. Osteochondral lesion with intra-fragmentary fracture (*black arrows*) after sustaining trauma. In such cases, fixation with 2 smaller fixation devices can be considered.

Lesion Factors

Lesion factors are crucial for determining if fixation is possible as well as choosing the fixation technique. Fragmentous OLT come in many shapes and sizes and may show a high heterogeneity in their morphologic presentation (see **Figs. 1–3**). One of the most important aspects is the lesion and fragment dimensions. A consensus statement from the International Consensus Group on Cartilage Repair of the Ankle recommends a minimum fragment diameter of 10 mm and bony thickness of 3 mm.[4] In practice, smaller diameter lesions are fixable but may require specific (smaller) fixation devices and may be less suited for surgeons who have limited experience with fixation of OLT.[27,28] Purely cartilaginous lesions may be considered for fixation but are stated to be unlikely to yield a successful outcome.[4] It is therefore crucial that surgeons have planned a "bail-out" option, in the form of an alternative surgical treatment, during preoperative planning in case of failed fixation intra-operatively.[3]

Another important aspect for the indication of fixation for OLT is the chronicity (see **Fig. 2**). In case of an acute osteochondral fracture, immediate fixation is indicated, as primary osteosynthesis resulting from compression yields good healing results without the need for additional subchondral augmentation by means of debridement or autologous bone grafting.[29] Additionally, in patients with a displaced fragment, immediate fixation may prevent further joint damage.[4] Lastly, surgeons should consider the presence of an intra-fragmentous fracture (see **Fig. 3**), which makes fixation of the fragment prone to failure, especially if one of the fragments is too small for fixation with a single fixation device. In case of a large fragment with a smaller fragment resulting from an intra-fragment fracture, surgeons should consider local excision and treatment (eg, with debridement and bone marrow stimulation [BMS] or scaffolding) of the smallest fragment and fixating the larger fragment in order to retain as much native cartilage as possible. It should be stated, however, that the results of such alternative fixation techniques are not known in the literature. Lastly, surgeons should incorporate the whole lesion morphology into their treatment plan. For example, in case of a (large) sub-fragmentous cyst (see **Fig. 2A**), surgeons may want to consider filling it with autologous spongious bone grafting.

Patient Factors

Patient factors influencing surgical outcomes should always be incorporated into the treatment plan. First, in skeletally immature patients without closed physis, an open treatment by means of an osteotomy is contraindicated when compromising the physis, which could lead to deformities.[15] In such cases, access can be possible arthroscopically or by means of arthrotomy. Secondly, patients with advanced ankle osteoarthritis (ie, advanced joint space narrowing or complete joint space obliteration), active or low-grade infections of the ankle joint, and patients medically unfit for surgery should not be treated with fixation. Additionally, from the authors' clinical experience, patients with a high body mass index (BMI) (>30) may have a higher susceptibility for non-union after fixation and should therefore be carefully considered. Moreover, other patient factors influencing union outcomes such as smoking, uncontrolled diabetes, and compliance with postoperative protocols should be considered when opting for a fixation procedure.[30] Lastly, any concomitant injury, such as lateral ankle instability, syndesmotic instability, fractures, or impingement, should be addressed in the treatment plan, as these are frequently encountered concomitantly to an OLT.[18–20]

In summary, a fixation procedure is indicated for the following lesion types.

- Symptomatic acute (<6 weeks symptoms) osteochondral fracture with a fragment amendable for fixation.

- Symptomatic non-acute primary osteochondral lesion with a fragment amendable for fixation not responsive to a minimum 3 to 6 months of conservative treatment.
- Non-primary symptomatic osteochondral lesion with a fragment amendable for fixation. However, these are only eligible if good-quality articular cartilage coverage of the fragment is present, as determined by preoperative MRI.

CONSERVATIVE TREATMENT AND PRE-HABILITATION

As stated earlier, in all cases of symptomatic chronic fragmentous OLT, conservative therapy should be considered for a minimum of 3 to 6 months. Conservative therapy consists of, or a combination of, the following strategies: activity modification, physical therapy, insoles, bracing in case of instability, weight-loss, or injections with hyaluronic acid.[3,31] Patients without symptoms or mild symptoms (ie, minimal interference of ankle complaints with activities of daily living or sports) may consider conservative therapy with yearly radiological evaluation, and as an alternative to surgery. Additionally, from the authors' clinical experience, conservative treatment of fragmentous OLT may result in union of the fragment in selected cases, such as in an acute on chronic injury.[32]

In patients who do not benefit from conservative therapy, and for whom surgical treatment is indicated, an individualized pre-habilitation protocol can be prescribed. Such a pre-habilitation program aims to optimize the preoperative physical well-being (eg, weight reduction, smoking cessation, and/or improving cardiovascular health) and ankle status. Examples of improving preoperative ankle status include strengthening the foot and ankle musculature and balance in patients with strength and balance deficits. Additionally, passive and active range of motion or stretching in patients with movement restrictions may be improved. Such pre-habilitation protocols have not been studied in foot and ankle patients but are supported by evidence from evidence of ACL-reconstructions.[33,34]

TECHNIQUES

The theoretic advantages of fixation are the preservation of the native hyaline cartilage, high-quality subchondral bone repair, and immediate stabilization of the fragment with restoration of the joint congruency.[7,8] Clinically, an important advantage is that prior fixation does not preclude any other surgical treatment in case fixation fails.

Surgical Approach

Both open and arthroscopic approaches for the fixation of OLT have been described.[7,9,10,15,27,35–37] Most literature has focused on the open approach via an osteotomy or arthrotomy, see **Figs. 4** and **6**.[7,9,10,15,27,35–37]

However, arthroscopic fixation is possible and described both in technique papers as well as clinical series.[7,11,35,38,39] Its theoretic advantage is the relatively less invasiveness over an open approach, see **Fig. 5**.

An important aspect when considering the surgical approach is the access to the lesion, which in turn is largely mediated by the lesion location. In case of lesions located more anteriorly, arthroscopic fixation is a good option as this is a less invasive technique.[7,35] It must be stated, however, that most lesions are located on the posteromedial talar dome and may be out of reach arthroscopically.[40,41] Adequate exposure to the lesion site is crucial for proper screw placement perpendicular to the fragment and articulating surface. Proper screw placement is important for sufficient

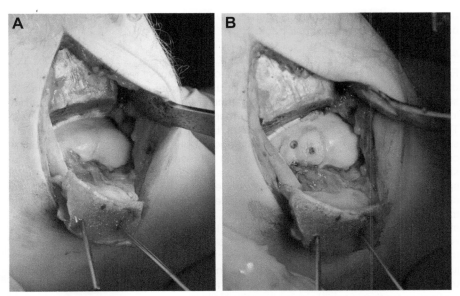

Fig. 4. Open fixation of an osteochondral fragment through a medial malleolar osteotomy approach. (*A*) Lesion in situ pre-fixation. (*B*) Status after fixation with 2 bio-absorbable screws to provide both compression and rotational stability.

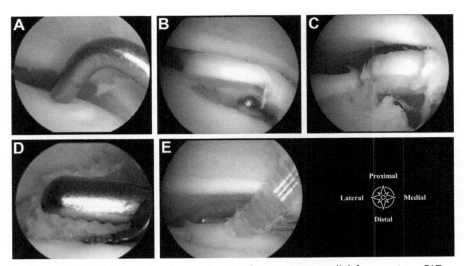

Fig. 5. Surgical technique of arthroscopic LDFF for an anteromedial fragmentous OLT according to Kerkhoffs and colleagues[7] Inspection and identification of the OLT. Lift (*A*), with a probe lifting the fragment (*B*). Drill, debridement, and drilling of the subchondral bone until healthy bone (*C*). Fill, filling of the debrided lesion site with autologous bone graft from the distal tibia (*D*). Fix, arthroscopic fixation using a bio-absorbable screw while stabilizing the fragment with a probe in order to avoid rotation during fixation (*E*).

compression and biomechanical stability, which may prevent the development of osteolytic changes in the screw track.[42]

Biologics and Adjuncts

From a biological perspective, acute lesions do not warrant biological adjuncts in aid of subchondral bone healing and fragment union. Acute on chronic and chronic lesions, however, can be seen as an intra-articular non-union, which may warrant biological adjectives in order to facilitate further healing and subchondral bone repair. This can be aided by means of debridement, bone marrow stimulation of the sclerotic subchondral bone, and transplanting autologous bone into the debrided site.[15] Especially in cases where a sub-fragmentous cyst is present (more common in chronic lesions), there may be a practical need for transporting additional cancellous and/or spongious bone in order to fill the debrided cyst in order to achieve adequate compression. The lift-drill-fill-fix (LDFF) procedure combines these aspects in order to facilitate the optimal healing environment, and can therefore be seen as an intra-articular non-union repair for these types of lesions.[7,15] An important technical note is that one should not overstuff the lesion site as this may prevent the restoration of the joint congruency and may adversely alter the joint biomechanics.[15] Biological adjuncts such as platelet-rich plasma or bone marrow aspirate concentrate have been utilized in ankle cartilage surgery with varying outcomes, and could be considered for fixation for their possible union benefits.[43,44] However, no evidence exists for their added benefit for OLT fixation to date.

Fixation Devices

An important topic of discussion in the fixation of OLT is the use of various fixation devices, which range from conventional cortical screws and bioabsorbable screws, to the smaller diameter Chondral Darts (Arthrex Inc., USA), poly-L-lactide pins (GRAND FIX, Depuy), and bone pegs.[9,14,15,36,37] Ideally, fragments are to be fixed using 2 screws or devices in order to give axial and rotational stability.[4,15] It is important that the choice of the fixation device is tailored to a specific lesion and fragment as they come in many shapes and sizes. The goal of choosing the ideal fixation device is to choose the option which provides the most biomechanical stability and compression as well as minimizing the chance of compromising the structural integrity of the fragment.[4,15] Practical reasons for choosing a certain device include experience of the surgeon, economic feasibility, access to the lesion, and product availability. For larger (>15 mm) fragments, self-tapping cortical screws or bioabsorbable screws will suffice. The devices are available in 2.0 mm and 2.7 mm diameters. An important technical note with conventional screws is to sink its head 0.5 mm to 1.0 mm below the articular cartilage surface in order to prevent chondral damage on the opposing side of the joint.[15] Intermediate size (10–15 mm) fragments can be fixed with 2 smaller fixation devices or a single screw. For smaller (<10 mm) fragments, bone pegs are the first-choice fixation device as a number of studies have shown good and reliable results with few union complications, which may be rooted in its adequate sizing and biological superiority as an autologous bone peg is used, see **Fig. 6**.[10,14,28,37]

It is also important to consider the thickness of the fragment, wherein the surgeon may opt for a smaller fixation device in thinner (<3 mm–see **Fig. 2B**) lesions, in order to prevent fracturing the fragment intra-operatively. Given the high variety in both fixation devices as well as their indications, no formal comparisons of their efficacy have been published in the literature. Surgeons are therefore advised to consider each device in the light of their specific case, including the earlier mentioned patient and lesion factors in their treatment choice.

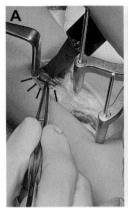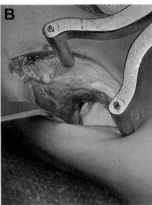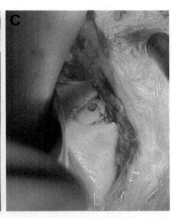

Fig. 6. (*A*) Fixation of an osteochondral fragment using a bone peg (*arrows*) harvested from the distal tibia through an anteromedial arthrotomy and Hintermann spreader. (*B*) In situ osteochondral lesion after circumferential cutting and "Lift,"" "Drill&" "Fill" phases. (*C*) Appreciation of the fixed osteochondral fragment using a bone peg.

AFTER TREATMENT AND FOLLOW-UP

After treatment following fixation of OLT varies throughout the literature, and is dependent on the surgical approach as well as the use of an osteotomy.[10,12,15,27,36,39] Most studies recommend an initial period of non–weight bearing by means of casting and crutches ranging from 4 to 6 weeks, which may be followed by a period of partial weight bearing and no peak forces up until 6 months postoperatively.[10,12,15,27,36,39] In any case, it is crucial that majority (>50%) union of the fragment has been achieved, without signs of fragment instability, screw protrusion, or osteotomy delayed/non-union (in case of osteotomy), before a patient is allowed to return to full weight-bearing activities. This should be assessed with follow-up imaging, such as a CT-scan after the periods of non- and partial weight bearing (**Fig. 7**). Clinicians may want to consider an additional period of partial weight bearing by means of a walker boot in case of a delayed or sub-optimal partial (<50%) union of the fixed fragment. In all cases, a personalized rehabilitation program led by an experienced foot and ankle physiotherapist is to be started as soon as possible with a strong cooperation between the treating physician and physiotherapist.[7,36] This program should focus on a step-wise approach of regaining full range of motion, foot and ankle strength, balance and proprioception, regaining a normal walking pattern, and return to work and sports.

The authors recommend intensive follow-up in the initial phase of wound healing, fragment union, and early rehabilitation in order to guide optimal after-treatment. A suggested timeline based on the literature would be initial wound healing phase (2 week postoperative visit for removal of stiches and revision of non–weight-bearing cast applied postoperatively), non–weight-bearing phase (from 0 to 4–6 week postoperatively, hereafter visit for non–weight-bearing cast removal and application of walking cast or walker), and partial weight-bearing phase (from 4–6 weeks postoperatively up to 8–12 weeks, hereafter removal of walking cast and imaging for assessment of fragment union and/or osteotomy union). Hereafter, postoperative visits at 6 months and 1 year follow-up are advised to guide the rehabilitation process and return to sports. Additionally, it is advised to follow up patients with CT-imaging or MR-imaging at 1 year postoperatively to assess fragment healing.[15,36]

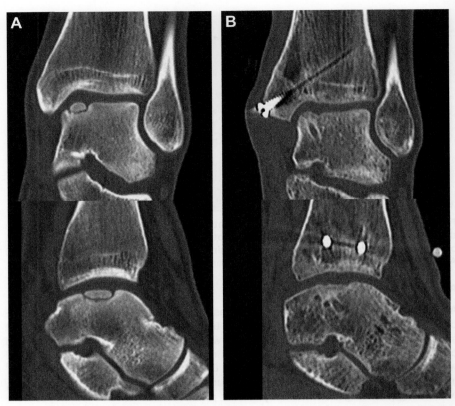

Fig. 7. Preoperative (*A*) and 1-year postoperative (*B*) CT-scan after open Lift-Drill-Fill-Fix. Complete fragment union. The bio-absorbable screw is partially resorbed.

OUTCOMES
Arthroscopic Fixation

Arthroscopic fixation of OLT was first described by Nakagawa and colleagues[35] Later, surgical technique additions were made by Kim and colleagues[38] and Kerkhoffs and-colleagues[7] In terms of outcomes for arthroscopic fixation, scant data are available.[7,11,35,38,39] The largest series to date is of the group from Kerkhoffs and colleagues describing a cohort of patients treated with arthroscopic LDFF.[7,11,39] In their 2020 paper describing 27 ankles, the afore-mentioned author group found that patients showed significantly improved clinical outcomes, by means of improved pain scores, functional outcomes (American Orthopedic Foot and Ankle Society Score [AOFAS] and the Foot and Ankle Outcome Score [FAOS]), and quality of life up to 2-year follow-up.[39] One patient received a revision surgery due to residual complaints. In terms of radiological outcomes, the authors observed that 92% of the patients had fragment union on 1-year follow-up CT-scans. In the same cohort, the authors observed superior subchondral bone healing compared to a cohort of patients treated with arthroscopic BMS, pointing to the advantages of the subchondral bone repair with autologous bone grafting.[8] In a recent paper describing the long-term outcomes of arthroscopic LDFF at an average of 7-year follow-up for 20 ankles, the authors observed that the afore-mentioned clinical outcomes to sustain over time, with a survival rate of the procedure of 87%. Though arthroscopic fixation can be considered technically challenging and few lesions are candidates for an arthroscopic approach due to their anterior location, arthroscopic fixation remains an attractive option as it allows for a minimally invasive approach with good results. Future studies will have to compare arthroscopic fixation with an open approach in order to substantiate the evidence-based treatment algorithm for fixation of OLT.

Open Fixation

Fixation of OLT through an open approach, including an arthrotomy or osteotomy, has been well described in the literature, though varies in the devices used.[9,10,12,14,27–29,36,37] From the current literature, it is known that open fixation yields good clinical outcomes up to mid-term follow-up and a significant improvement of clinical and functional outcomes.[9,10,12,14,27–29,36,37] At long-term follow-up, limited though promising results are available.[10,29]

The most commonly used fixation device is a bioabsorbable screw or conventional screw. Choi and colleagues,[36] utilizing bioabsorbable screws in 26 ankles observed a significant improvement in the visual analog scale (VAS) for pain and Foot Function Index at an average 28 months postoperatively, with 5 patients undergoing revision surgery. Rikken and colleagues,[15] in their recent surgical technique and results of 15 ankles undergoing open LDFF with bio-absorbable or conventional screws, found a significant improvement in the numeric rating scale for pain during walking, rest, and running, and the FAOS and AOFAS at 2-year follow-up compared to the baseline. The authors reported 1 revision surgery. Schuh and colleagues,[9] treating 20 ankles with K-wire fixation for fragmentous OLT, found good to excellent results in all patients at an average 46-month follow-up.

A number of the papers on clinical outcomes concern the outcomes from bone peg fixation.[10,14,28] Kumai and colleagues[10] observed good outcomes in 89% of their 27 ankles at an average 7-year follow-up. Haraguchi and colleagues,[14] with their series of 45 ankles who underwent bone peg fixation, found that the Japanese Society for Surgery of the Foot ankle/hindfoot scale improved significantly from 63.5 points preoperatively to 93.0 postoperatively, and observed 1 treatment failure. Park and colleagues,[28] who included 25 ankles, observed an improvement in the VAS score for pain and AOFAS score from 6.3 and 70.6 preoperatively to 1.6 and 91.1 at a mean 22-month follow-up, respectively. Other studies focused on the use of poly-L-lactide pins.[12,27] Nakasa and colleagues observed superior clinical outcomes in 36 ankles fixed with poly-L-lactide pins through an open approach, even with smaller (<100 mm^2) OLT, compared to arthroscopic BMS. The aforementioned authors observed a mean postoperative AOFAS score of 97.3 out of 100 points.

In terms of radiological outcomes, it can be observed that fragment union is to be achieved in 77% up to 100% of cases.[9,10,12,14,15,27,28,36,37] Interestingly, Choi and colleagues[36] found an irregular margin and low density of the fragment on preoperative CT-scanning to be significantly associated with non-union. This is further substantiated by the findings from Nakasa and colleagues[12] who observed bone marrow lesions in the group with most bone resorption in the fixed fragment as measured with preoperative CT-scanning. Theoretically, this could be an important clue for the success of fragment fixation in OLT as the more biomaterial is available, in the form of viable bone, the higher chance there could be for successful union. Adding autologous bone, and therefore seeing the fixation procedure of a chronic fragmentous OLT as an intra-articular non-union repair, may improve the biological environment as well as the subchondral healing.[7] Due to the limited number of patients reported in the literature, no formal comparison is available on the optimal cutoff lesion dimensions for successful fixation, and the current guidelines are therefore based on expert opinion.[4]

WHAT TO DO IN FAILURE CASES?

A failed fixation for OLT does not preclude any follow-up surgical treatment for the OLT. This makes a wide range of surgical options available for the OLT which includes BMS, autologous or allogenic (osteo) chondral transplantation, or regenerative treatments.[1,3] Follow-up treatment should be chosen based on the optimal patient and lesion characteristics as outlined by the current evidence.[3] It is important, however, to determine what the origin of the failure is, namely if this concerns a radiological non-union (with or without complaints) or concerns recurrent symptoms from the OLT after union. In case of asymptomatic non-union without symptoms of locking (ie, no grossly instable fragment), no protruding fixation material, and no symptomatic loose bodies, clinicians can choose with their patients to treat this with supervised neglect and periodized imaging. In case of symptomatic non-union or recurrent symptoms from the OLT, the earlier mentioned surgical treatment options and non-operative treatment may be considered. Another scenario which should be considered is when a screw or fixation device is protruding from a fragment with union. In such cases, the screw should be removed in order to prevent damage to the joint. Lastly, refixation can only be considered in cases of fragments with good-quality overlying articular cartilage, which should be assessed preoperatively with MRI and intra-operatively as well. In case the cartilage is of insufficient quality as assessed intra-operatively, another surgical treatment should be available as a "bail-out" option.

CLINICS CARE POINTS

- Symptomatic acute or chronic fragmentous OLT should always be considered for in situ fixation.
- Pre-treatment imaging, by means of CT scanning or MR imaging, is helpful in clinical decision-making.
- Lesion and patient characteristics guide the treatment algorithm for fixation of fragmentous OLT.
- Choice of type and number of screws, or alternative fixation methods, is based on lesion and fragment morphology, size, and thickness, and should ideally be with 2 screws or pins or pegs in order to provide axial and rotational stability.
- Fixation of OLT can be through an arthroscopic or open approach and yields good clinical outcomes with union rates ranging from 77% to 100%.
- If fixation fails and/or results in a symptomatic non-union or malunion, all other surgical cartilage treatments for OLT are still feasible.

DISCLOSURE

Work performed at the Department of Orthopedic Surgery and Sports Medicine, Amsterdam UMC, Location AMC, Amsterdam, The Netherlands.

FINANCIAL STATEMENT

No funding was received for this study.

ACKNOWLEDGMENTS

The authors thank Dr Jari Dahmen for his assistance in drafting this article, Dr Sjoerd AS Stufkens for his clinical input, and acknowledge the shared work from the Amsterdam Ankle Cartilage Team in preparing this article.

REFERENCES

1. Lambers KTA, Dahmen J, Reilingh ML, et al. No superior surgical treatment for secondary osteochondral defects of the talus. Knee Surgery, Sport Traumatol Arthrosc 2018;26:2158–70.
2. Dahmen J, Lambers KTA, Reilingh ML, et al. No superior treatment for primary osteochondral defects of the talus. Knee Surg Sport Traumatol Arthrosc 2018; 26:2142–57.
3. Rikken QG, Kerkhoffs GM. Osteochondral Lesions of the Talus: An Individualized Treatment Paradigm from the Amsterdam Perspective. Foot Ankle Clin 2021; 26(1):121–36.
4. Reilingh ML, Murawski CD, DiGiovanni CW, et al. Fixation Techniques: Proceedings of the International Consensus Meeting on Cartilage Repair of the Ankle. Foot Ankle Int 2018;39(1_suppl):23S–7S.
5. Ramponi L, Yasui Y, Murawski CD, et al. Lesion Size Is a Predictor of Clinical Outcomes after Bone Marrow Stimulation for Osteochondral Lesions of the Talus: A Systematic Review. Am J Sports Med 2017;45(7):1698–705.
6. Shimozono Y, Donders JCE, Yasui Y, et al. Effect of the Containment Type on Clinical Outcomes in Osteochondral Lesions of the Talus Treated With Autologous Osteochondral Transplantation. Am J Sports Med 2018;46(9):2096–102.
7. Kerkhoffs GMMJ, Reilingh ML, Gerards RM, et al. Lift, drill, fill and fix (LDFF): a new arthroscopic treatment for talar osteochondral defects. Knee Surgery, Sport Traumatol Arthrosc 2016;24(4):1265–71.
8. Reilingh ML, Lambers KTA, Dahmen J, et al. The subchondral bone healing after fixation of an osteochondral talar defect is superior in comparison with microfracture. Knee Surgery, Sport Traumatol Arthrosc 2018;26(3):2177–82.
9. Schuh A, Salminen S, Zeiler G, et al. Ergebnisse der refixation der osteochondrosis dissecans des talus mit kirschnerdrähten. Zentralbl Chir 2004;129(6):470–5.
10. Kumai T, Takakura Y, Kitada C, et al. Fixation of osteochondral lesions of the talus using cortical bone pegs. J Bone Jt Surg - Ser B 2002;84(3):369–74.
11. Rikken QGH, Altink JN, Dahmen J, et al. Sustained clinical success at 7-year follow-up after arthroscopic Lift-Drill-Fill-Fix (LDFF) of primary osteochondral lesions of the talus. Knee Surgery, Sport Traumatol Arthrosc 2023. https://doi.org/10.1007/s00167-022-07243-5.
12. Nakasa T, Ikuta Y, Ota Y, et al. Clinical Results of Bioabsorbable Pin Fixation Relative to the Bone Condition for Osteochondral Lesion of the Talus. Foot Ankle Int 2019;40(12):1388–96.
13. Sawa M, Nakasa T, Ikuta Y, et al. Outcome of autologous bone grafting with preservation of articular cartilage to treat osteochondral lesions of the talus with large associated subchondral cysts. Bone Jt J 2018;100B(5):590–5.
14. Haraguchi N, Shiratsuchi T, Ota K, et al. Fixation of the osteochondral talar fragment yields good results regardless of lesion size or chronicity. Knee Surgery, Sport Traumatol Arthrosc 2020;28(1):291–7.
15. Rikken QGH, Favier BJC, Dahmen J, et al. Open Lift-Drill-Fill-Fix for Medial Osteochondral Lesions of the Talus: Surgical Technique. Oper Orthop Traumatol 2023. Accepted.

16. Hintermann B, Regazzoni P, Lampert C, et al. Arthroscopic findings in acute fractures of the ankle. J Bone Joint Surg Br 2000;82(3):345–51. http://www.ncbi.nlm.nih.gov/pubmed/10813167.

17. Hintermann B, Boss A, Schäfer D. Arthroscopic findings in patients with chronic ankle instability. Am J Sports Med 2002;30(3):402–9.

18. Martijn HA, Lambers KTA, Dahmen J, et al. High incidence of (osteo)chondral lesions in ankle fractures. Knee Surgery, Sport Traumatol Arthrosc 2020;0123456789. https://doi.org/10.1007/s00167-020-06187-y.

19. Wijnhoud EJ, Rikken QGH, Dahmen J, et al. One in Three Patients With Chronic Lateral Ankle Instability Has a Cartilage Lesion. Am J Sports Med 2022. https://doi.org/10.1177/03635465221084365.

20. Dahmen J, Jaddi S, Hagemeijer NC, et al. Incidence of (Osteo)Chondral Lesions of the Ankle in Isolated Syndesmotic Injuries: A Systematic Review and Meta-Analysis. Cartilage 2022;13(2). https://doi.org/10.1177/19476035221102569.

21. Rikken QGH, Wolsink LME, Dahmen J, et al. 15% of Talar Osteochondral Lesions Are Present Bilaterally While Only 1 in 3 Bilateral Lesions Are Bilaterally Symptomatic. J Bone Jt Surg Am 2022;00:1–9.

22. Verhagen RAW, Maas M, Dijkgraaf MGW, et al. Prospective study on diagnostic strategies in osteochondral lesions of the talus. Is MRI superior to helical CT? J Bone Joint Surg Br 2005;87(1):41–6.

23. Nakasa T, Ikuta Y, Yoshikawa M, et al. Added Value of Preoperative Computed Tomography for Determining Cartilage Degeneration in Patients With Osteochondral Lesions of the Talar Dome. Am J Sports Med 2018;46(1):208–16.

24. Yasui Y, Hannon CP, Fraser EJ, et al. Lesion Size Measured on MRI Does Not Accurately Reflect Arthroscopic Measurement in Talar Osteochondral Lesions. Orthop J Sport Med 2019;7(2). https://doi.org/10.1177/2325967118825261.

25. Raikin SM, Elias I, Zoga AC, et al. Osteochondral lesions of the talus: Localization and morphologic data from 424 patients using a novel anatomical grid scheme. Foot Ankle Int 2007;28(2):154–61.

26. Cohen MM, Vela ND, Levine JE, et al. Validating a New Computed Tomography Atlas for Grading Ankle Osteoarthritis. J Foot Ankle Surg 2015;54(2):207–13.

27. Nakasa T, Ikuta Y, Sumii J, et al. Clinical Outcomes of Osteochondral Fragment Fixation Versus Microfracture Even for Small Osteochondral Lesions of the Talus. Am J Sports Med 2022;50(11):3019–27.

28. Park CH, Song KS, Kim JR, et al. Retrospective evaluation of outcomes of bone peg fixation for osteochondral lesion of the talus. Bone Joint J 2020;102(10):1349–53.

29. Dunlap BJ, Ferkel RD, Applegate GR. The "LIFT" lesion: Lateral inverted osteochondral fracture of the talus. Arthroscopy 2013;29(11):1826–33.

30. Jensen SS, Jensen NM, Gundtoft PH, et al. Risk factors for nonunion following surgically managed, traumatic, diaphyseal fractures: a systematic review and meta-analysis. EFORT Open Rev 2022;7(7):516–25.

31. Di Gesù M, Fusco A, Vetro A, et al. Clinical effects of image-guided hyaluronate injections for the osteochondral lesions of ankle in sport active population. J Sports Med Phys Fitness 2016;56(11):1339–45.

32. Aalders MB, Dahmen J, Kerkhoffs GMMJ. Trauma-induced spontaneous union of a talar osteochondritis dissecans: case report. J ISAKOS 2023;8(4):261–6.

33. Cunha J, Solomon DJ. ACL Prehabilitation Improves Postoperative Strength and Motion and Return to Sport in Athletes. Arthrosc Sport Med Rehabil 2022;4(1):e65–9.

34. Shaarani SR, O'Hare C, Quinn A, et al. Effect of Prehabilitation on the Outcome of Anterior Cruciate Ligament Reconstruction. Am J Sports Med 2013;41(9):2117–27.
35. Nakagawa S, Hara K, Minami G, et al. Arthroscopic fixation technique for osteochondral lesions of the talus. Foot Ankle Int 2010;31(11):1025–7.
36. Rak Choi Y, Soo Kim B, Kim YM, et al. Internal Fixation of Osteochondral Lesion of the Talus Involving a Large Bone Fragment. Am J Sports Med 2021;49(4):1031–9.
37. Park CH, Choi CH. A novel method using bone peg fixation for acute osteochondral fracture of the talus: a surgical technique. Arch Orthop Trauma Surg 2019;139(2):197–202.
38. Kim HN, Kim GL, Park JY, et al. Fixation of a Posteromedial Osteochondral Lesion of the Talus Using a Three-Portal Posterior Arthroscopic Technique. J Foot Ankle Surg 2013;52(3):402–5.
39. Lambers KTA, Dahmen J, Reilingh ML, et al. Arthroscopic lift, drill, fill and fix (LDFF) is an effective treatment option for primary talar osteochondral defects. Knee Surgery, Sport Traumatol Arthrosc 2020;28(1):141–7.
40. van Diepen PR, Dahmen J, Altink JN, et al. Location Distribution of 2,087 Osteochondral Lesions of the Talus. Cartilage 2020. https://doi.org/10.1177/1947603520954510. 194760352095451.
41. Van Bergen CJA, Tuijthof GJM, Maas M, et al. Arthroscopic accessibility of the talus quantified by computed tomography simulation. Am J Sports Med 2012;40(10):2318–24.
42. Nakasa T, Ikuta Y, Tsuyuguchi Y, et al. MRI Tracking of the Effect of Bioabsorbable Pins on Bone Marrow Edema After Fixation of the Osteochondral Fragment in the Talus. Foot Ankle Int 2019;40(3):323–9.
43. Xie X, Zhang C, Tuan RS. Biology of platelet-rich plasma and its clinical application in cartilage repair. Arthritis Res Ther 2014;16(1):1–15.
44. Dombrowski ME, Yasui Y, Murawski CD, et al. Conservative Management and Biological Treatment Strategies: Proceedings of the International Consensus Meeting on Cartilage Repair of the Ankle. Foot Ankle Int 2018;39(1_suppl):9S–15S.

Regeneration
Bone-Marrow Stimulation of the Talus—Limits and Goals

Jeff S. Kimball, MD[1], Richard D. Ferkel, MD[2], Eric I. Ferkel, MD*

KEYWORDS

- Ankle arthroscopy • Bone marrow stimulation • Cartilage • Osteochondral lesion
- Microfracture • Talus

KEY POINTS

- Bone Marrow Stimulation should be used for lesions <100 to 107.4 mm^2 in area.
- Bone Marrow Stimulation < 5 mm in depth.
- Bone Marrow Stimulation should be used with concomitant cartilage restoration techniques in lesions 15 mm in diameter or greater.
- Biologic adjuvants have been shown to improve patient outcomes when performing bone marrow stimulation procedures.
- Optimal surgical management will depend on the location and size of the lesion, chronicity, and presence of cystic component.

INTRODUCTION/BACKGROUND

Articular cartilage is quintessential in facilitating the smooth and painless mechanical motion of joints. Osteochondral lesions and degenerating articular cartilage have long been a difficult challenge for the musculoskeletal surgeon. Because of its histologic structure and susceptibility to injury from shear forces, cartilage regeneration remains a difficult enigma in joint preservation. The quest for cartilage regeneration has taken many forms, one of the earliest techniques, that remains a mainstay in many treatments today, is bone marrow stimulation. As early as the 1950s, Pridie described methods for accessing bone marrow contents for cartilage regeneration with some success[1,2] These early techniques were intended to create a joint resurfacing in the setting of osteoarthritis and involved open subchondral drilling.

Department of Orthopaedic Surgery, Southern California Orthopedic Institute, Van Nuys, CA, USA
[1] Present address: 341 Magnolia Avenue, #101, Corona, CA 92563.
[2] Present address: 6815 Noble Avenue, Suite 200, Van Nuys, CA 91405.
* Corresponding author. 6815 Noble Avenue, Suite 200, Van Nuys, CA 91405.
E-mail address: eferkel@scoi.com

Foot Ankle Clin N Am 29 (2024) 281–290
https://doi.org/10.1016/j.fcl.2024.01.001
1083-7515/24/© 2024 Elsevier Inc. All rights reserved.

foot.theclinics.com

Later, more minimally invasive approaches were pioneered with the use of arthroscopy. During the 1980s, Lanny Johnson developed the concept of abrasion arthroplasty to try to regrow articular cartilage.[3] Subsequently in 2001, the traditional "microfracture" technique was popularized by Richard Steadman using an ice pick type instrument for subchondral penetration.[4] This technique used angled "picks" or awls of varying angles to allow easy access to any articular surface. Around the same era with the advent of the arthroscopic shaver, abrasion arthroplasty also gained favor. The surgical goal of each of these procedures was to create a perpendicular penetration in the subchondral bone exposing the cartilage defect to the marrow elements including growth factors and progenitor cells. These elements were then attracted to the area of fracture where a marrow clot would form allowing the proliferation of cells into what we now know to be a fibrocartilaginous tissue, somewhat similar in appearance and function to the native hyaline cartilage.

While osteochondral lesions can cause disability and pain in any synovial joint, the focus of this discussion will be on osteochondral lesions of the ankle which present an important pathology that causes significant morbidity and cost annually.

Etiology & Incidence

Osteochondral lesions of the talus (OLT) occur in up to 6.5% of ankle sprains or fractures with up to 98% of lateral and 70% of medial osteochondral defects the result of trauma to the ankle.[5–7] There is a male predominance demonstrating a 6.9 times increased risk for development compared to females in the second decade of life.[8] Bilateral OLT occur in 10% to 15% of patients with a significantly larger defect present on the more symptomatic side.[9,10] The biomechanics of the ankle at its location under near total body weight in the upright posture lead to significant forces across the joint that are multiplied many times with running and rotational injuries.[11] The talar side of this joint is at particularly high risk of injury due to its comparatively softer cartilage compared to the opposing distal tibial cartilage.[12] This leads to a predominance of lesions localized to the anterolateral or posteromedial talar dome.[13,14] Aside from trauma-related etiologies, OLT can also occur as a result of vascular insufficiency, primary osteonecrosis, or genetic predisposition.[8,15]

Diagnosis

Initial patient evaluation requires a thorough history and physical examination. Symptomatology may include pain and swelling, stiffness, and/or mechanical symptoms. Point tenderness near the area of a lesion is also common. OLTs often present with vague nonspecific symptoms, often with global ankle pain, and often in combination with swelling or subjective catching sensation in the joint. Diagnosis is made with weight-bearing plain 3-view radiographic examination of the ankle and to rule out other associated pathology that may be contributing to pain. Osteochondral lesions are often not visible on plain view radiographs and confirmatory diagnosis may require MRI or computed tomography (CT) scans. Earlier stage lesions may benefit from MRI evaluation to further delineate the bone marrow edema that occurs in earlier stages and is associated with a painful OLT. MRI has proven a useful tool in evaluating osteochondral lesions of the talus.[16] It is important to note however that MRI has also been shown to overestimate the size of the OLT compared to arthroscopic evaluation.[17] In older more chronic lesions, a CT scan is a useful preoperative planning tool to better quantify the amount of bone involvement in the defect and can assist with operative decision making.

If an osteochondral lesion is suspected or seen on imaging, it is essential to confirm that the lesion is in fact the source of the patient's pain. Osteochondral lesions can notoriously be asymptomatic thus exclusion of other pathology is essential. Consideration can be given to a diagnostic injection for confirmation. Asymptomatic lesions are common and should not be treated surgically.[9,10]

Once a symptomatic osteochondral lesion is verified as the primary source of the patient's symptoms, a treatment strategy can be devised. Understanding the patient's activity goals and setting appropriate expectations is critical for success.

Treatment of OLT can vary based on the chronicity, size, location, and depth of the lesion. Acute injuries are sometimes amenable to repair if an osseus base is large enough and remains attached to the articular cartilage.[18] If the lesion is not repairable, bone marrow stimulation techniques are considered. If the lesion is too large for bone marrow stimulation, then one must consider the ever-growing list of approaches to surgical management of OLT.[19] This review will focus on bone marrow stimulation to support cartilage regeneration.

DISCUSSION
Bone Marrow Stimulation as a Surgical Approach to Osteochondrial Lesions of the Talus

While there are several techniques to penetrate the subchondral bone with varying depth, prior surface preparation is critical to having a successful outcome. Steadman and colleagues described the importance of height of the cartilage rim surrounding the lesion.[20] If there is not adequate surrounding cartilage rim height, then the marrow clot will dissipate and the localized cell reaction cannot proceed. This is the foundational concept as to why bone marrow stimulation shows less favorable outcomes when used in the degenerative joint with thin remaining cartilage surrounding the full thickness lesions.

The 2 predominating techniques used in bone marrow stimulation today include awl puncture and drilling. Each has its merits and pitfalls. Awl penetration avoids the potential heat-induced cell damage caused by drilling but may not penetrate to an adequate depth. When using an awl, the author uses a 1–2 mm awl placing holes 3–4 mm apart with a depth of 2–4 mm. Critical to awl penetration is to avoid placing the holes too close or to penetrate too deeply as this can lead to subchondral plate collapse. A variety of awl shapes with varying tip angles can facilitate treatment in difficult to reach locations. A potentially negative aspect of awl penetration is the cone-like shape of the tip leading to widening of the hole as the awl goes deeper. Because of this, the use of an awl in both animal and human models has been associated with compacted bone and increased osteocyte necrosis.[21]

Microfracture technique may contribute to a deterioration of the subchondral bone architecture which may ultimately limit clinical outcomes due to a more rapid degradation of the resulting fibrocartilage over time (**Figs. 1** and **2**).[22]

Drilling can be done with smaller diameter wires, 0.035 inch (0.9 mm) or 0.045 inch (1.1 mm) trocar tipped Kirschner wires with uniform diameter. The Depth of penetration is also an important component with drilling offering greater access to deeper marrow elements which may lead to superior cartilage repair.[21] The depth of penetration has more recently become a topic of significant importance. Chen and colleagues reported that drilling to 6 mm produced better fill and quality of cartilage than the traditional 2 mm depth.[23] However, when drilling was limited to 2 mm, results were similar to those of traditional awl bone marrow stimulation (**Fig. 3**).

While drilling may be the preferred method for bone marrow stimulation, the lesion location can render drilling too difficult or can increase the procedure morbidity. Transmalleolar drilling can be done but it does violate the intact tibial plafond articular

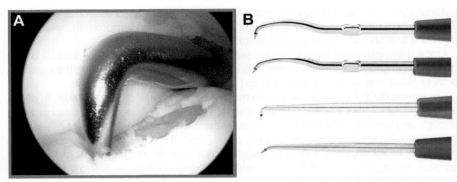

Fig. 1. Microfracture of an OLT (*A*) Use of an angled awl for bone marrow stimulation of a medial talar dome osteochondral lesion in the right ankle. Visualization is from the postero-lateral portal. (*B*) Various awl shapes to facilitate access to difficult to reach articular zones.

cartilage. Instead, trans-talar drilling can be done to access the talus. In some cases, curved awls can offer more surgeon and patient friendly access in difficult to reach locations.

Lastly, a newer technology utilizing a bone marrow stimulation curved delivery device (SmartShot, Marrow Access Technologies, Eden Prairie, MN) with a 1 mm diameter stainless steel needle allows for accessing more challenging areas of the talus or

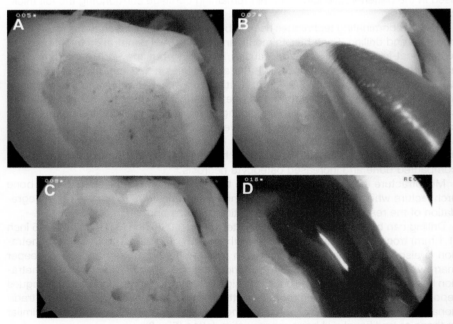

Fig. 2. Microfracture of an osteochondral lesion (*A*) OLT after lesion debridement and cartilage side wall preparation, (*B*) Awl penetration of subchondral bone of OLT, (*C*) Demonstration of awl puncture holes through subchondral plate, (*D*) Marrow clot forming a "Crimson Duvet" over the area of OLT.

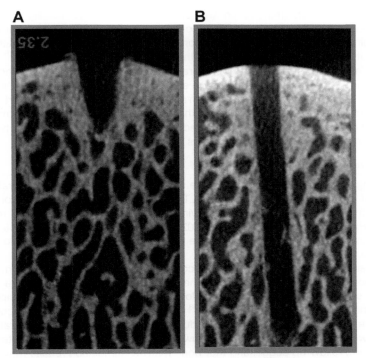

Fig. 3. Microfracture versus drilling (*A*) Microscopic representation of cone-shaped awl penetration of subchondral plate. (*B*) Microscopic representation of wire penetration of subchondral plate.

tibial plafond with 6 mm depth penetration. A recent study showed that the needle-puncture devices preserved "underlying subchondral bone relative to other marrow access approaches."The benefit of this device is less bone damage, less compaction, no heat generation to allow for better marrow access, and potentially better bone remodeling (**Fig. 4**).

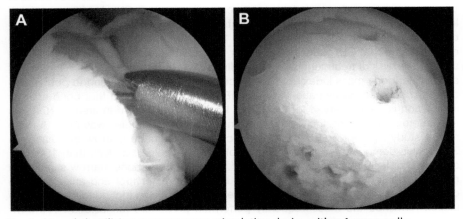

Fig. 4. (*A and B*) Utilizing marrow access stimulation device with a 1-mm needle.

OLT in children can often present with an intact cartilage layer but significant bone marrow edema and subchondral cystic changes. In these cases, retrograde trans-talar drilling can offer a reasonable option to stimulate bone marrow contents with or without a bone graft without violating the tenuous overlying cartilage.[24,25]

The senior authors' preferred postoperative course when treating OLT includes a compressive dressing and postoperative splint. The splint and stitches are removed at 10 to 14 days and the patient is placed in a removable splint to allow the start of range of motion and strengthening exercises. If the lesion size was less than 100 mm^2, then a course of non-weight bearing is maintained for 2 to 4 weeks. For larger lesions greater than 100 mm^2, non weight bearings status is implemented for 4 to 6 weeks.

Clinical Outcomes

A growing number of long-term outcome studies have demonstrated favorable outcomes of bone marrow stimulation for OLTs. Corr and colleagues reported on 45 patients with 10 to 12 year follow-up showing a 93% survival rate and 86% return to sport.[26] Park and colleagues evaluated 202 ankles clinical and reported 97% survival rate for lesions of less than 150 mm^2 size with stable clinical results at 10 to 19 year follow-up.[27]

A systematic review by Kerkhoffs and colleagues evaluating 323 ankles in 319 patients showed a mean postoperative American Orthopedic Foot and Ankle Society (AOFAS) score of 84 at mean 13 year follow-up with 78% of patients participating in sports and only a 7% reoperation rate.[28] These long-term studies are encouraging that bone marrow stimulation is an enduring and effective treatment strategy for OLT. However, Ferkel and colleagues showed that 35% of patient results deteriorated at long-term follow-up suggesting that bone marrow stimulation results may worsen over time in some patients.[29]

Recently biologic agents have become a popular adjuvant to further improve upon these promising long-term study results. Recent studies have shown that biologic agents such as Platelet-Rich Plasma (PRP), Bone Marrow Aspirate Concentrate (BMAC), Hyaluronic Acid (HA), and scaffold-based therapies provide favorable improvement in the treatment of OLT.[30–32] These agents require further study but are the frontier of a growing movement in cartilage regenerative medicine.

Limits

Subchondral bone loss and large defect size are the greatest limiting factors related to bone marrow stimulation as a viable treatment option for OLT. Chuckpaiwong and colleagues suggested that a cutoff point exists for risk of clinical failure with an osteochondral defect area of approximately 10 × 15 mm.[33] Several studies have demonstrated that OLT defect size greater than approximately 150 mm^2 by MRI are at increased risk of treatment failure, as defined by AOFAS score <80.[33–35] Increasing age, higher body mass index, and presence of osteophytes also lead to poorer outcomes.[33] A recent systematic review of 1868 ankles suggested that bone marrow stimulation is best reserved for OLT sizes less than 107.4 mm^2 in area or 10.2 mm in diameter.[36] However, the level of evidence from these studies was poor. A more recent study by Park and colleagues which evaluated bone marrow stimulation in 202 ankles demonstrated a survival rate of 97% for lesion size less than 150 mm^2 and 83% for lesions greater than 150 mm^2.[27] Furthermore, bone marrow stimulation remains an internationally trusted technique in the greater foot and ankle surgeon community. A study by Guelfi and colleagues in 2021 showed that bone marrow stimulation remained the most frequently performed procedure for lesions >150 mm^2 based on a survey of 1804 surgeons from 80 countries.[37]

Lesion containment is also an important limiting factor; talus shoulder lesions, which are uncontained lesions, demonstrate worse clinical outcomes.[38] In the same study, contained lesions faired equally better whether located medial or lateral. Similarly, the presence of subchondral bone cysts has been reported to correlate with worse clinical outcomes. Cheng and colleagues demonstrated that subchondral cysts with cutoff values of area of 90 mm^2, a depth of 7.56 mm, or a volume of 428 mm^3 produced a negative effect on clinical outcomes after bone marrow stimulation for OLT.[39]

In a recent consensus meeting, bone grafting was recommended for cystic lesions greater than 5 mm of depth (grade of evidence of E, 77% agreed, strong consensus).[40,41]

SUMMARY

Bone marrow stimulation technique and indications have evolved since its inception. Today awl or wire penetration techniques are used primarily. When used for treatment of osteochondral lesions of the talus, it has demonstrated good clinical outcomes with appropriate patient and lesion selection. However, studies vary on the long-term durability of the fibrocartilage.

CLINICS CARE POINTS

- Bone marrow stimulation technique has evolved over time with the evidence most strongly supporting awl penetration or drilling with a 0.045-mm wire to 6 mm depth.
- Intact cartilage rim surrounding the osteochondral lesion with maintained height is critical to contain marrow clot after stimulation.
- Biologic adjuvants can improve outcomes of bone marrow stimulation techniques.
- Bone marrow stimulation in the ankle remains an important and useful treatment strategy for osteochondral lesions of sizes less than 107.4 mm^2 in area or 10.2 mm in diameter.

DISCLOSURE

J.S. Kimball - No Disclosures. R.D. Ferkel - Arthrex, Inc: Other financial or material support; Arthroscopy Association of North America: Board or committee member; Cannuflow: Paid consultant; Geistlich Pharma: Paid consultant; Mitek: Other financial or material support; Sawbones/Pacific Research Laboratories: IP royalties; Smith & Nephew: IP royalties; Other financial or material support; Paid consultantVericel: Paid consultant; Wolters Kluwer Health - Lippincott Williams & Wilkins: Editorial or governing board; Publishing royalties, financial or material support. E.I. Ferkel - AAOS: Board or committee member; American Orthopaedic Foot and Ankle Society: Board or committee member; American Orthopaedic Society for Sports Medicine: Board or committee member; Arthrex, Inc: Paid consultant; Paid presenter or speaker; Arthroscopy Association of North America: Board or committee member; DJ Orthopaedics: Research support; Ferring Pharmaceuticals: Paid consultant; Paid presenter or speaker; Medartis: Paid consultant; Mitek: Paid consultant; Research support; Ossio: Paid consultant; Ossur: Research support; Smith & Nephew: Paid consultant; Research support.

REFERENCES

1. Pridie K. A method of resurfacing osteoarthritic knee joint. J Bone J Surg Br 1959; 41:618–9.

2. Insall J. The Pridie debridement operation for osteoarthritis of the knee. Clin Orthop Relat Res 1974;101:61–7.
3. Friedman MJ, Berasi CC, Fox JM, et al. Preliminary results with abrasion arthroplasty in the osteoarthritic knee. Clin Orthop Relat Res 1984;182:200–5.
4. Steadman JR, Rodkey WG, Rodrigo JJ. Microfracture: surgical technique and rehabilitation to treat chondral defects. Clin Orthop Relat Res 2001;(391 Suppl):S362–9.
5. Zwingmann J, Sudkamp NP, Schmal H, et al. Surgical treatment of osteochondritis dissecans of the talus: a systematic review. Arch Orthop Trauma Surg 2012; 132(9):1241–50.
6. Flick AB, Gould N. Osteochondritis dissecans of the talus (transchondral fractures of the talus): review of the literature and new surgical approach for medial dome lesions. Foot Ankle 1985;5(4):165–85.
7. Verhagen RA, Struijs PA, Bossuyt PM, et al. Systematic review of treatment strategies for osteochondral defects of the talar dome. Foot Ankle Clin 2003;8(2): 233–42, viii-ix.
8. Bruns J, Habermann C, Werner M. Osteochondral lesions of the talus: a review on talus osteochondral injuries, including osteochondritis dissecans. Cartilage 2021; 13(1_suppl):1380S–401S.
9. Hermanson E, Ferkel RD. Bilateral osteochondral lesions of the talus. Foot Ankle Int 2009;30(8):723–7.
10. Rikken QGH, Wolsink LME, Dahmen J, et al. 15% of talar osteochondral lesions are present bilaterally while only 1 in 3 bilateral lesions are bilaterally symptomatic. J Bone Joint Surg Am 2022;104(18):1605–13.
11. Procter P, Paul JP. Ankle joint biomechanics. J Biomech 1982;15(9):627–34.
12. Athanasiou KA, Niederauer GG, Schenck RC Jr. Biomechanical topography of human ankle cartilage. Ann Biomed Eng 1995;23(5):697–704.
13. van Dijk CN, Reilingh ML, Zengerink M, et al. Osteochondral defects in the ankle: why painful? Knee Surg Sports Traumatol Arthrosc 2010;18(5):570–80.
14. Zengerink M, Struijs PA, Tol JL, et al. Treatment of osteochondral lesions of the talus: a systematic review. Knee Surg Sports Traumatol Arthrosc 2010;18(2): 238–46.
15. Stattin EL, Wiklund F, Lindblom K, et al. A missense mutation in the aggrecan C-type lectin domain disrupts extracellular matrix interactions and causes dominant familial osteochondritis dissecans. Am J Hum Genet 2010;86(2):126–37.
16. Mintz DN, Tashjian GS, Connell DA, et al. Osteochondral lesions of the talus: a new magnetic resonance grading system with arthroscopic correlation. Arthroscopy 2003;19(4):353–9.
17. Yasui Y, Hannon CP, Fraser EJ, et al. Lesion size measured on MRI does not accurately reflect arthroscopic measurement in talar osteochondral lesions. Orthop J Sports Med 2019;7(2). 2325967118825261.
18. Kerkhoffs GM, Reilingh ML, Gerards RM, et al. Lift, drill, fill and fix (LDFF): a new arthroscopic treatment for talar osteochondral defects. Knee Surg Sports Traumatol Arthrosc 2016;24(4):1265–71.
19. Shimozono Y, Vannini F, Ferkel RD, et al. Restorative procedures for articular cartilage in the ankle: state-of-the-art review. Journal of ISAKOS 2019;4(5):270–84.
20. Steadman JR, Rodkey WG, Briggs KK. Microfracture: its history and experience of the developing surgeon. Cartilage 2010;1(2):78–86.
21. Kraeutler MJ, Aliberti GM, Scillia AJ, et al. Microfracture versus drilling of articular cartilage defects: a systematic review of the basic science evidence. Orthop J Sports Med 2020;8(8). 2325967120945313.

22. Shimozono Y, Coale M, Yasui Y, et al. Subchondral bone degradation after microfracture for osteochondral lesions of the talus: an mri analysis. Am J Sports Med 2018;46(3):642–8.

23. Chen H, Hoemann CD, Sun J, et al. Depth of subchondral perforation influences the outcome of bone marrow stimulation cartilage repair. J Orthop Res 2011; 29(8):1178–84.

24. Carlson MJ, Antkowiak TT, Larsen NJ, et al. Arthroscopic treatment of osteochondral lesions of the talus in a pediatric population: a minimum 2-year follow-up. Am J Sports Med 2020;48(8):1989–98.

25. Dahmen J, Steman JAH, Buck TMF, et al. Treatment of osteochondral lesions of the talus in the skeletally immature population: a systematic review. J Pediatr Orthop 2022;42(8):e852–60.

26. Corr D, Raikin J, O'Neil J, et al. Long-term outcomes of microfracture for treatment of osteochondral lesions of the talus. Foot Ankle Int 2021;42(7):833–40.

27. Park JH, Park KH, Cho JY, et al. Bone marrow stimulation for osteochondral lesions of the talus: are clinical outcomes maintained 10 years later? Am J Sports Med 2021;49(5):1220–6.

28. Rikken QGH, Dahmen J, Stufkens SAS, et al. Satisfactory long-term clinical outcomes after bone marrow stimulation of osteochondral lesions of the talus. Knee Surg Sports Traumatol Arthrosc 2021;29(11):3525–33.

29. Ferkel RD, Zanotti RM, Komenda GA, et al. Arthroscopic treatment of chronic osteochondral lesions of the talus: long-term results. Am J Sports Med 2008;36(9): 1750–62.

30. Yasui Y, Wollstein A, Murawski CD, et al. Operative treatment for osteochondral lesions of the talus: biologics and scaffold-based therapy. Cartilage 2017; 8(1):42–9.

31. Migliorini F, Eschweiler J, Goetze C, et al. Cell therapies for chondral defects of the talus: a systematic review. J Orthop Surg Res 2022;17(1):308.

32. Seow D, Ubillus HA, Azam MT, et al. Limited evidence of adjuvant biologics with bone marrow stimulation for the treatment of osteochondral lesion of the talus: a systematic review. Knee Surg Sports Traumatol Arthrosc 2022;30(12):4238–49.

33. Chuckpaiwong B, Berkson EM, Theodore GH. Microfracture for osteochondral lesions of the ankle: outcome analysis and outcome predictors of 105 cases. Arthroscopy 2008;24(1):106–12.

34. Choi WJ, Park KK, Kim BS, et al. Osteochondral lesion of the talus: is there a critical defect size for poor outcome? Am J Sports Med 2009;37(10):1974–80.

35. Guo QW, Hu YL, Jiao C, et al. Arthroscopic treatment for osteochondral lesions of the talus: analysis of outcome predictors. Chin Med J (Engl) 2010;123(3): 296–300.

36. Ramponi L, Yasui Y, Murawski CD, et al. Lesion Size Is a Predictor of Clinical Outcomes After Bone Marrow Stimulation for Osteochondral Lesions of the Talus: A Systematic Review. Am J Sports Med 2017;45(7):1698–705.

37. Guelfi M, DiGiovanni CW, Calder J, et al. Large variation in management of talar osteochondral lesions among foot and ankle surgeons: results from an international survey. Knee Surg Sports Traumatol Arthrosc 2021;29(5):1593–603.

38. Choi WJ, Choi GW, Kim JS, et al. Prognostic significance of the containment and location of osteochondral lesions of the talus: independent adverse outcomes associated with uncontained lesions of the talar shoulder. Am J Sports Med 2013;41(1):126–33.

39. Cheng X, Su T, Fan X, et al. Concomitant subchondral bone cysts negatively affect clinical outcomes following arthroscopic bone marrow stimulation for osteo-chondral lesions of the talus. Arthroscopy 2023;39(10):2191–9.e1.

40. Hannon CP, Bayer S, Murawski CD, et al. Debridement, Curettage, and Bone Marrow Stimulation: Proceedings of the International Consensus Meeting on Cartilage Repair of the Ankle. Foot Ankle Int 2018;39(1_suppl):16S–22S.

41. Zlotnick HM, Locke RC, Stoeckl BD, et al. Marked differences in local bone re-modelling in response to different marrow stimulation techniques in a large ani-mal. Eur Cell Mater 2021;41:546–57.

Regeneration
AT-AMIC Technique: Limits and Indication

Camilla Maccario, MD, Agustín Barbero, MD, Cristian Indino, MD*

KEYWORDS

- AT-AMIC • AMIC • OLT • Osteochondral lesion of the talus • Cartilage
- Ankle arthroscopy

KEY POINTS

- Good data for osteochondral lesion of the talus (OLT) are still missing. Multicentric database and registry could support a better understanding and an improved algorithm of treatment.
- Arthroscopic autologous matrix-induced chondrogenesis (AT-AMIC) is a reliable all-arthroscopic one-step technique for OLT treatment.
- Proper joint distraction allows successful AT-AMIC for most of the OLT, regardless of size and location.
- Body mass index, age, size, and location of the lesion are the main prognostic factors.
- Recent imaging developing suggests integrating MRI with weight-bearing computed tomography scan. Milan-Tel Aviv protocol has been designed to improve the decision-making process.

 Video content accompanies this article at http://www.foot.theclinics.com.

INTRODUCTION
Definition

Several acronyms have been developed and used for cartilage lesion. In 2018, the International Consensus Meeting on Cartilage Repair of the Ankle developed an agreement on terminology (level of Evidence E)[1]: the definition "chondral lesion" is referred to an isolated chondral damage, "subchondral bone lesion" is referred to isolated bone lesion, and "osteochondral lesion of the talus (OLT)" is the appropriate definition for a combined osseous and chondral lesion.

Although the main cause for OLT is posttraumatic, not every patient is able to recall a traumatic event in his history. However, not all the lesions are symptomatic.

Ankle and Foot Unit, Humanitas San Pio X, Via Francesco Nava 31, Milano
* Corresponding author. Via Francesco Nava 31, 20159, Milan, Italy.
E-mail address: cristian.indino@gmail.com

Foot Ankle Clin N Am 29 (2024) 291–305
https://doi.org/10.1016/j.fcl.2023.07.008
1083-7515/24/© 2023 Elsevier Inc. All rights reserved.

Patient perception of the pathologic condition and of the treatment and the algorithm of treatment itself are still under debate. Good-quality high-volume data collection could help in the future to address these questions and define the role of reference centers.

Bone and/or Cartilage, Where Is the Real Problem?

Amsterdam Ankle Cartilage Group recently went deep into the "Cascade" of events from ankle sprain or fracture (first step), passing through the "invisible" cartilage crack (second step) causing the osteochondral lesion (third step) that may end up in ankle arthritis on-set (fourth step).[2] Furthermore, they described as "accidental findings" the asymptomatic ones, "acute" the symptomatic within 6 weeks from trauma and symptoms on-set, "chronic" if symptoms have been referred for longer than 6 weeks, and "acute on chronic" when lesions become symptomatic after a trauma but they where are there before.

A consensus on the appropriate treatment is missing. It may be correlated to the lack of understanding of the pathologic condition but also to the extremely fast evolution of products and devices, often driven from marketing opportunity rather than scientific data analysis.

During the last decades, several surgical procedures have been proposed for OLT treatment, claiming good to excellent result at short follow-up: osteochondral autograft transfer system (OATS)/mosaicplasty, osteochondral allografts, autologous chondrocyte implantation (ACI, MACI), matrix-associated stem cell transplantation (MAST), osteochondral scaffold (Maioregen; Fin-Ceramica Faenza SpA, Italy), and juvenile cartilage allograft transplantation. Unfortunately, diversity is not always good for science.

Different scaffolds, membranes, biological technologies, and support are constantly introduced into "OLT market." Hence, we are facing increasing costs, and worldwide heterogeneity due to both costs and regulatory processes, without good, high-volume and long-term data.

Author's Opinion: "Treat the Patient and Not the Lesion!"

Bad-looking OLT on MRI could behave as accidental findings. Small lesions could have a strong impact on quality life of patients. The combination of recent imaging evolution and higher interest in patient-related outcomes may be the key to better understand the pathology, and its positive and negative predictors of outcomes.

Imaging

Surgeons used to rely typically on x-rays, MRI, and computed tomography (CT) scan. Each of these tools has a specific role in the evaluation of OLTs.

- *X-rays:* They are not useful to identify the OLTs that are often missed on standard radiographs. Weight-bearing x-rays are important to identify any ankle or foot malalignment that should be addressed together with the treatment of OLT.
- *MRI:* It is used to assess ankle cartilage, detect bone marrow edema, or diagnose concomitant soft tissue pathologic conditions.[3] It can overestimate the lesion size when bone edema is present. Together with CT scan, MRI is the most common diagnostic tools used, with high sensitivity and specificity (**Fig. 1**).
- *CT scan:* CT scan is used to assess the bony morphology and better estimate the size of OLT[3] (**Fig. 2**).

Parallel to this standard diagnostic setting, weight-bearing CT scan (WBCT) could significantly improve the preoperative and postoperative analyses of this pathologic

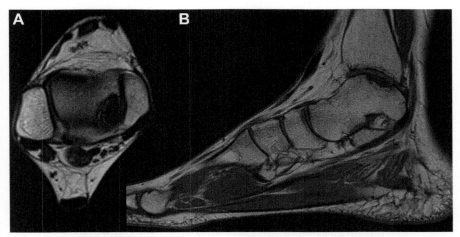

Fig. 1. MRI of a preoperative patient with an OLT located in zones 4 and 7 of Raikin zones. (*A*) Axial view. (*B*) Sagittal view.

condition as well as for other foot and ankle pathologic conditions.[4,5] A more recent feature includes semiautomated algorithms capable of measuring angles, creating a visual representation of the anatomic axis of the bones, and obtaining distance maps of the relative distance between 2 articular surfaces.

Semiautomatic distance mapping has been previously proven to be relatable to a force platform analysis,[6] making the WBCT a tool, which can provide functional analysis too.

Since this finding, our imaging protocol shifted from an MRI-based one to a more comprehensive one. The Milan-Tel Aviv protocol comprises a biological and mechanical lesion assessment (**Fig. 3**).

- The biological assessment relies on traditional MRI imaging. It assesses the lesion morphology, location, and the presence of bone edema allowing to

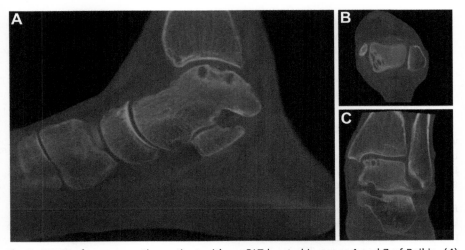

Fig. 2. WBCT of a preoperative patient with an OLT located in zones 4 and 7 of Raikin. (*A*) Sagittal view. (*B*) Axial view. (*C*) Coronal view.

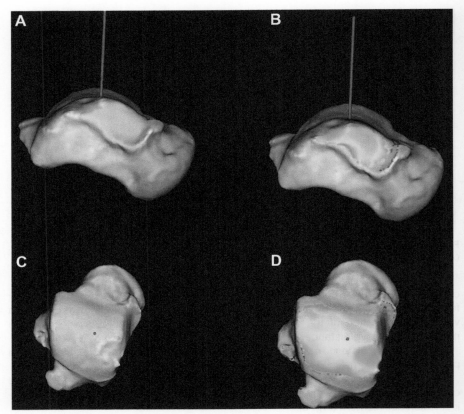

Fig. 3. (*A*) Sagittal view. (*B*) Sagittal view with distance mapping (DM). (*C*) Axial view. (*D*): Axial view with DM. Red line in sagittal and red dot in axial represent the position of the axis of the tibia calculated by semiautomated manner.

distinguish between biologically active lesions (with bone edema) and biological inactive lesions (without bone edema).

- The preoperative and postoperative mechanical evaluations of the lesion are assessed with WBCT: They allow identifying patients with altered pattern of contact pressure on and around the OLT (biomechanically active lesions) and patients with normal contact pressure distribution despite OLT (biomechanically inactive lesions).

Combining the data between MRI and WBCT will open a new scenario in which OLT will be categorized not only about size, depth, and dimensions but also about a combination of biomechanics and biologic activity of the lesion (**Table 1**). Future investigations about this topic will correlate these features with the outcomes of the treatments and will provide a more reliable solution to the complex problem of OLT.

Patient-reported outcome scores
Understanding the patient's perception of pain and loss of function is essential to the preoperative and postoperative analyses. Currently, most physicians rely on patient-reported outcome scores (PROMS): they comprise a validated series of questions given to the patients throughout their treatment that, sometimes, deal with general

Table 1
Milan-Tel Aviv protocol of imaging setting of osteochondral lesions of the talus

| | | Weight-bearing CT Scan Distance Mapping at the Lesion Site | |
		Altered Pattern	Normal Pattern
Bone edema on MRI	Present	Biological and biomechanically active	Biological active and biomechanically inactive
	Absent	Biomechanically active and biological inactive	Biological and biomechanically inactive

health status and not with foot and ankle health. Physicians and researchers can use the data to evaluate the patient's status and improvement. However, many authors have discussed the limitations of PROMS as a reliable source of information.[7] Palmen and colleagues[8] have discussed the low patient compliance rate and the inability to provide a long-term follow-up (citation). Czerwonka and colleagues[9] have discussed that many patients need help understanding the questions, and therefore, the answers given are biased (citation). Other authors discussed the potential bias of targeting specific patient groups with access to higher levels of health-care systems, and finally, authors have described the effect of filling the questioner in a stressful environment on the accuracy of the patient answers (operating room or doctor's office).[9] This raises the question, why, in an era where data are gathered electronically, are we still using pen and paper to collect data about patient status? What is the value of asking a patient in Europe if he can walk a New York block when phone-apps are actively measuring the number of steps we take daily? Moreover, why do we need to ask awkward questions about social interactions when most patients report their social experiences on social media platforms? The evolution in patient follow-up will require modifying the currently used PROMS to a system that need good and high-volume data and that will mine data from the patient in a more reliable and up-to-date manner.

Driving Factors for Surgery

Key performance indicators that drive patients toward surgery are as follows:

- *Symptoms*: If patient is asymptomatic, no surgery is needed.
- *Time*: Acute lesions should be approached as soon as possible, most of all with fixation, if possible. If it is not an acute problem, then surgery should be planned after 6 months of conservative treatment failures.
- *Patient's predictors of outcomes*: Body max index (BMI), age, expectations, and compliance.
- *Lesions predictors of outcomes:* Size, location, depth, and revision.

Amsterdam Ankle Cartilage Group proved that fixation should be pursued as first option regardless of the onset of the lesion (acute or chronic) but depending on the presence of a fixable subchondral bone fragment (at least 10 mm in width and 3 mm in depth)[3] the lift, drill, fill and fix concept (LDFF). When LDFF is not a viable option, all arthroscopic autologous matrix-induced chondrogenesis (AT-AMIC) is our choice of procedure.[10]

AMIC consists of bone marrow stimulation (BMS) via microfracture, optional structural support via autograft application for filling the defective area, and application of potentially chondrogenic scaffolds (collagen types I/III bilayer matrix). It has the advantages of being a single-step (unlike ACI/MACI), less-expensive (unlike ACI/MACI or allograft applications) procedure[11,12] and avoids knee-related donor site morbidity, which is a major concern for OATS.[12–16]

AMIC combines the biological power of BMS with a suitable membrane that enhances the chondrogenic differentiation of mesenchymal stem cells. This wealthy healing environment stimulates chondrocytes to enhance proteoglycan deposition.[17,18] Herein, the clot formed because of hemorrhage is covered and stabilized.

AT-AMIC differ from AMIC because is a totally arthroscopic technique without any osteotomy.

INDICATIONS

1. Symptomatic not-fixable chronic osteochondral lesion of the talus of types III and IV according to Berndt and Harty's classification[19] confirmed by clinical examination, MRI, and CT scan.
2. Ankle pain for more than 6 months or trauma occurred more than 6 months ago that does not respond to conservative treatment.
3. Skeletal maturity but described even for symptomatic juvenile osteochondral lesion.[20]
4. Primary or revision procedure.

CONTRAINDICATIONS

1. Ankle arthritis
2. Noncorrectable hindfoot malalignment
3. Infection
4. Metabolic arthropathy
5. Systemic disorders

Kissing lesions should not be considered as an absolute contraindication because addressing the major lesion could improve ankle function and reduce symptomatology.

Moreover, ankle and foot malalignment should be considered a relative contraindication: AT-AMIC is a mini-invasive all-arthroscopic technique that can be associated to realignment procedure, thus allowing to expand indication for joint preserving surgery even in case of misaligned ankle with symptomatic OLT.

AT-AMIC: SURGICAL TECHNIQUE

The entire procedure is performed arthroscopically in supine position using standard anteromedial and anterolateral portals, with application of a thigh tourniquet (Video 1).

After the arthroscopic inspection of the joint, the presence of the defect should be confirmed, as well as its size and shape. At this point, a Hintermann spreader (Integra LifeSciences, Plainsboro, NJ) is percutaneously placed to distract the joint and allow exposure of the lesion, avoiding the use of a traction (**Fig. 4**). The Hintermann spreader has an opening lever arm applied on two 2.5-mm K-wires previously positioned in the tibia and talar bone medially or laterally, according to the lesion side. In the case of a lateral lesion, care must be taken to insert the proximal K-wire in the tibial bone, avoiding the fibula, to achieve better distraction.

After identification of the lesion, the damaged cartilage and the necrotic bone is removed with an arthroscopic curette to create a regular-shaped site (**Fig. 5**A). Microfractures are induced by a Chondro Pick (Arthrex, Naples, FL) on the healthy subchondral bone underneath the defect (**Fig. 5**B). To measure the lesion, a preoperative size is measure on CT-scan and confirmed intraoperatively using a probe. At this point, a 5.5-mm cannula is inserted through the closest portal to the lesion. The intra-articular water is removed and the Chondro-Gide matrix Geistlich Pharma AG (Geistlich Surgery, Wolhusen, Switzerland), previously prepared according to the sizing, is

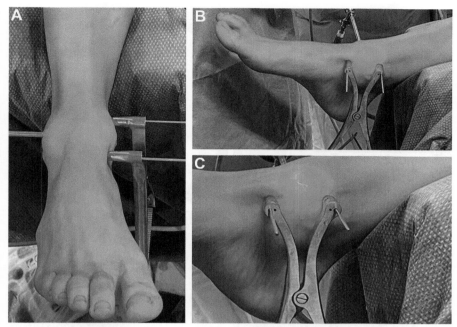

Fig. 4. Medial positioning of the Hintermann's spreader. The proximal pin is located in the distal tibia and the distal pin goes to the talus in order to generate working space after distraction. (*A*) Anteroposterior view of the ankle in the surgical field with the Hintermann's spreader medial positioning. (*B*) Medial view of the ankle in the same context. (*C*) Zoom in of the medial view image.

inserted through the cannula, and positioned at the lesion site (**Fig. 5**C). If needed, autologous bone graft arthroscopically harvested form anterior wall of tibia can be used to fill bone defects below the cartilage layer. Slightly downsizing the membrane is advisable because it has the trend to be slightly oversized once introduced in a wet environment. Signing the top of the membrane with a dermographic pen before the implantation allows avoiding membrane upside-down positioning.

Once the matrix fits the lesion, it is glued by fibrin glue (Tisseel; Baxter, Deerfield, IL). The Hintermann spreader is removed, and the stability of the matrix within a normal ankle range of motion is then arthroscopically checked.

Our postoperative management requires movement restriction for 15 days and no weight-bearing for 30 days.

RESULTS

In a systematic review and meta-analysis from 2021, with a total of 492 patients assessed,[21] the visual analogue scale (VAS) improved 4.6 points from baseline, American Orthopedic Foot and Ankle Society (AOFAS) score improved 32.47 points and foot function index (FFI) score significantly improved 30.93 points to the 3 to 5-year follow-up.

In a 5-year follow-up prospective cohort study[12] comparing AMIC to microfractures at a mean follow-up of 43.5 months, the AOFAS, VAS, and Tegner scores were greater

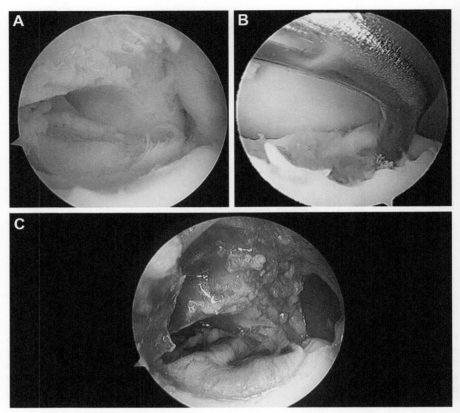

Fig. 5. Arthroscopic images from AMIC. (*A*) Regular shape after arthroscopic debridement. (*B*) Microfractures. (*C*) Membrane positioning.

in the AMIC group. The AMIC group evidenced lower rates of reoperation (P = .008) and failure (P = .003).

Return to Sport

Many patients ask to return to the same activity level they had before the onset of symptoms but the ideal treatment is controversial: we need to balance an early return to sport with the necessity of cartilage restoration with high-quality osteochondral tissue.[22]

In a retrospective observational cross-sectional study, Usuelli and colleagues[22] analyzed 26 consecutive patients who underwent surgical treatment of AT-AMIC with the aim of determining the rate of return of patients to sport. About 80.8% of the patients returned to the same preinjury sport. The mean follow-up was 42.6 months. Significant improvements were observed for AOFAS, SF-12, Halasi, and UCLA scores.

Moreover, prognostic factors we have to advice to the patient are described next.

Patient's Predictors of Outcomes

Age

In a retrospective study, D'Ambrosi and colleagues[18] evaluated 31 patients divides in 2 groups (younger and older than 33 years). They assessed VAS, AOFAS score, Short

Form 12 (SF-12) CT, and magnetic resonace imaging (MRI) in a follow-up of 6, 12, and 24 months. A significant improvement in all clinical parameters and a reduced lesion sized at final follow-up have been noticed: AT-AMIC can be considered a mini-invasive, safe, and reliable procedure that allows effective healing with a significant clinical improvement regardless of age and clinical results are related to starting conditions of the ankle.

In an attempt of answering the incognita of youth limit, in other study, Usuelli and colleagues[20] evaluated clinical and radiological outcomes of patients aged younger than 20 years treated with AT-AMIC: all clinical scores significantly improved and lesion area significantly reduced from 119.1 to 77.9 mm^2 as assessed by CT and from 132.2 to 85.3 mm^2 as assessed by MRI. Moreover, they noted an important correlation between intraoperative size of the lesion and BMI.

However, Kubosch and colleagues[16] in 2015 studied 17 patients and reported that patients aged 45 years and older showed significantly lower values concerning postoperative pain and higher values concerning overall contentment in comparison to patients less than 45 years with even better outcome parameters (AOFAS score, FFI, and Magnetic Resonance Observation of Cartilage Repair Tissue [MOCART] score). It needs to be considered that possible explanations for a better outcome in the subgroup of patients aged 45 years or older could be lower expectations in comparison to younger patients.

The opposite statement resulted in a study made by Migliorini and colleagues in 2022.[23] Regardless of including knee cartilage defects, they found that patient age had a negative association with the AOFAS score and Lysholm Knee Scoring Scale.

Body Mass Index

Kubosh and colleagues[16] found that patients with a BMI greater than 30 showed a significantly lower AOFAS score and a significantly higher VAS postoperative in comparison to patients with a BMI less than 30.

Similarly, D'Ambrosi and colleagues[24] evaluated 52 patients with chronic OLTs, and BMI, VAS, AFOAS score, and SF-12 were analyzed. A subanalysis dividing the talus into 6 areas was performed. In the central lesions, BMI was connected to the lesion size turning this into the first study to find a linear relationship between lesion size and BMI.

In another study, Usuelli and colleagues[25] assessed functional and radiographic outcomes in 37 patients after AT-AMIC in 2 weight groups with OLT regarding their BMI minor or greater than 25. The overweight group presented a significantly larger lesion measured with MRI; thereafter, the authors concluded that OLTs in overweight patients were characterized by a larger preoperative size. At final follow-up, both groups showed a significant clinical improvement, deducing that AT-AMIC can be considered a safe and reliable procedure, regardless of weight, with a significant improvement also in quality of life.

Usuelli and colleagues assessed that the higher is the BMI, the lower will be functional scores preoperatively and postoperatively with a delta of improvement linked to the standard population, who generally has high preop and postop scores.

Lesion Predictor of Outcomes

Size

When AT-AMIC emerged, the indication preference was for lesions greater than 150 mm^2 or revisions. Now, not only personal experience from the authors but also scientific literature[12,22,24,26] betray those confines, with published reports ranging from 1 up to

2 cm in diameter with no strong correlation between lesion size and functional outcome. In AMIC revision, the mean area of the defect is described even at 2.8 ± 1.9 cm^2.[27]

Usuelli and colleagues[24,25] demonstrated a significant correlation between BMI and lesion size and a significant impact of OLTs on quality of life.

Fueled by scientific literature, it seems to be than a high BMI combined with larger defects and concomitant chronic ankle instability has been found predictive of worse results in regards of functionality and postoperative pain level.[16,28]

Location

Most OLTs are found on the anterolateral or posteromedial talar dome[15,22] but the variability is noteworthy. Usuelli and colleagues analyzed 52 patients with symptomatic chronic OLTs[24] and they were located as follows: medial 20 (38.50%); central 13 (24.0%); and lateral 19 (36.50%); anterior 24 (46.15%); middle 16 (30.77%); and posterior 12 (23.08%). In the central group, the authors identified a negative correlation between aging and AOFAS and positive correlation between BMI and lesion size indicating that central lesions could be more likely worsened by increased BMI due to biomechanical overloading.

Although almost no difference between medial and lateral was found in Usuelli's study, Yontar and colleagues[14] found a huge proportion of their lesions positioned in the medial side. On the counterpart, Ayyaswamy and colleagues[15] found most of their patients to have a lesion on the lateral side.

In 2022, Richter and colleagues[29] studied one of the largest populations. They assessed 136 lesions in a prospective study at 5 years follow-up of AMIC plus Peripheral Blood Concentrate. Chondral lesions were located as follows: medial talar shoulder only, 62%; lateral talar shoulder only, 42%; medial and lateral talar shoulder, 7%; and tibia, 18%. They concluded that the follow-up parameters did not significantly differ between 2 and 5 years' follow-up including PROMS and MRI stage of the chondral lesions.

Bone marrow edema

Bone marrow edema lesions have been identified as structural changes of the subchondral bone and may represent the precursor of subchondral bone attrition or cartilage deterioration.[30] These identifiable lesions provide a challenge for treatment because the most clinically effective treatment remains unclear and various techniques have been investigated.[30] Even the anatomopathological significance of bone marrow edema is not yet clear: a characteristic MRI pattern includes a wide variety of histopathologic pictures, causal mechanisms, and prognosis.[31] D'Ambrosi and colleagues in 2016 confirmed the efficacy of AT-AMIC in the treatment of OLTs in patients with bone marrow edema with a significant reduction of lesion size at 2-year follow-up: they found that patient with bone marrow edema had a bigger lesion size at each follow-up concluding that edema has a correlation with the area of the lesion and that AT-AMIC acts on both OLT and bone marrow edema.[31]

Bone marrow edema may be filled with bone substitute or autogenous bone even in case of OLTs. Subchondroplasty has been recently proposed for OLT surgery[3]: calcium phosphate is injected via a retrograde approach to fill the subchondral lesion and may be combined with additional arthroscopic treatments of the OLT.[3] Only few short-term clinical outcomes are available for subchondroplasty for talar pathologic conditions. In case of unclear presence of OLT over talar bone marrow edema, we suggest to perform subchondroplasty under direct visualization of a 2-mm arthroscopic system (NanoScope, Arthrex, Naples, FL, USA) to check for any intra-articular leaking of calcium phosphate and to confirm the presence of OLT: in this case, nanoscopy should be converted in a standard arthroscopy to address it.

COMPLICATIONS

On a systematic review in 2022,[32] the rate of revision surgery and surgical failure of AMIC were 7.8% and 6.2%, respectively. As any other surgery, the fluctuation of complications is not only related to an excellent indication but to surgeon's learning curve.

Conversely, in a systematic review and meta-analysis, Valderrabano and colleagues in 2021[21] investigated 12 studies with a total of 323 patients. Regarding safety, there were only 6 patients who required a subsequent surgery within 5 years after the initial procedure. There were no reported adverse events or complications directly related to the AMIC procedure, whereas the 6 revision surgeries correspond to 1% of the treated patients. Importantly, no patients required conversion to ankle fusion or arthroplasty.

In a systematic review and meta-analysis of 2023 by Amsterdam UMC Group, matrix-assisted BMS represented the treatment of 1031 lesions out of 6261, with a complication rate of 3% that was the lowest rate among the other techniques (shared with cartilage implantation): superficial infection was the most occurring complication in the group.[33]

DISCUSSION

AMIC offers a way to incorporate the standard BMS, with addition biological features for larger lesions size.

AT-AMIC is a procedure improving AMIC with the advantage of an all-arthroscopic technique and the key factor in the articular distraction, through Hintermann spreader properly positioned.

A recent review suggested updating the 150 mm limit of microfractures[34–37] to 107.4 mm.[38] Authors agree with this principle, finding no restrictions for AT-AMIC for smaller lesions, rather than economics.

The role of BMI as a prognostic factor is significant and should not be left apart as an information provided to the patient.

Limits

As any other surgical technique, AT-AMIC is not flawless and has its own limitations.

- *Age*: Because it is a biological treatment, age in considered a limitation even if no differences were founded in some studies.
- *Malalignment*. It is a general limitation for every isolate cartilage treatment but AT-AMIC could be integrated in ankle malalignment procedures when OLT is present, limiting the invasiveness and morbidity of the procedure. Besides, it allows enlarging joint-preserving surgeries indications in case of ankle malalignments.
- *Lesion site*: The use of Hintermann's spreader allows reaching lesions in the anterior two-thirds of talar dome, whereas in lesions located in the posterior one-third of talus, different strategies or approaches should be considered.
- *Learning curve*: Finally, surgeons should have completed the learning curve for basic ankle arthroscopy procedures, before approaching AT-AMIC surgeries.

BIOLOGIC ADJUVANTS

Biological therapies represent an additional topic that should be consider as technology and research procedures. Platelet-rich plasma (PRP) and bone marrow aspirate concentrate are autologous blood products aiming at improving the quality of cartilage and subchondral bone repair.[3] Adipose tissue is another source of autologous stem cells.[39] These tools can be used in both conservative treatment and as augmentation for surgery.[40,41] Among the recent treatment described, MAST is a modification of AMIC with a potentially higher concentration of stem cells in the implanted matrix that is impregnated with stem cell-rich blood harvested from the pelvic bone: it showed encouraging results at 2-year follow-up.[42] Recently, a novel technique has been proposed: it consists of treating osteochondral lesions with debridement and autologous minced cartilage harvested from the border of the lesion mixed up with PRP and fixed with autologous thrombin solution (Autocart procedure, Arthrex, Munich, Germany).[43] It has been described also for ankle OLTs but clinical studies are expected to confirm its effectiveness. In the field of biological adjuvants, despite good and encouraging outcomes, the type of therapy, timing of use, and composition of treatments are mainly based on expert opinion, with limited high-level evidence in the literature.

CLINICS CARE POINTS

- The first surgery intention to treat an OLT should be fixation, if is not possible, the authors suggest AT-AMIC.
- Milano-Tel Aviv imaging protocol comprises a biological and mechanical lesion assessment introducing WBCT to OLT. This standpoint arises as a useful combination tool, defining biomechanics and biologic activity of the lesion.
- Proper joint distraction allows successful AT-AMIC for most of the OLT, regardless of size and location.
- Hintermann spreader is percutaneously placed to distract the joint and allow exposure of the lesion, avoiding the use of a traction using two 2.5-mm K-wires previously positioned in the tibia and talar bone medially or laterally.
- Biological therapies represent an additional topic that should be consider as technology and research procedures. Among them PRP, adipose tissue, and MAST have encouraging outcomes.

DISCLOSURE

The authors have no conflicts of interest to disclose.

ACKNOWLEDGMENTS

The authors would like to thank Federico G. Usuelli and Ben Efrima for their valuable contribution to this article.

SUPPLEMENTARY DATA

Supplementary data related to this article can be found online at https://doi.org/10.1016/j.fcl.2023.07.008.

REFERENCES

1. Murawski CD, Nunley JA, Pearce C, et al. Terminology for osteochondral lesions of the ankle: proceedings of the International Consensus Meeting on Cartilage Repair of the Ankle. J ISAKOS 2022;7(2):62–6.

2. Dahmen J, Karlsson J, Stufkens SAS, et al. The ankle cartilage cascade: incremental cartilage damage in the ankle joint. Knee Surg Sports Traumatol Arthrosc 2021; 29(11):3503–7 [Erratum in: Knee Surg Sports Traumatol Arthrosc. 2022;30(8): 2881].

3. Rikken QGH, Kerkhoffs GMMJ. Osteochondral Lesions of the Talus: An Individualized Treatment Paradigm from the Amsterdam Perspective. Foot Ankle Clin 2021;26(1):121–36.

4. de Cesar Netto C, Bang K, Mansur NS, et al. Multiplanar Semiautomatic Assessment of Foot and Ankle Offset in Adult Acquired Flatfoot Deformity. Foot Ankle Int 2020;41(7):839–48.

5. Efrima B, Barbero A, Ovadia JE, et al. Axial rotation analysis in total ankle arthroplasty using weight-bearing computer tomography and three-dimensional modeling. Foot Ankle Surg 2023. https://doi.org/10.1016/J.FAS.2023.05.001.

6. Efrima B, Barbero A, Ovadia JE, et al. Classification of the Os Calcis Subtalar Morphology in Symptomatic Flexible Pediatric Pes Planus Deformity Using Weightbearing CT and Distance Mapping. Foot Ankle Int 2023;44(4):322–9.

7. Bernstein DN, Jones CMC, Flemister AS, et al. Does Patient-Reported Outcome Measures Use at New Foot and Ankle Patient Clinic Visits Improve Patient Activation, Experience, and Satisfaction? Foot Ankle Int 2023. https://doi.org/10.1177/10711007231163119. 10711007231163119.

8. Palmen LN, Schrier JC, Scholten R, et al. Is it too early to move to full electronic PROM data collection?: A randomized controlled trial comparing PROM's after hallux valgus captured by e-mail, traditional mail and telephone. Foot Ankle Surg 2016;22(1):46–9.

9. Czerwonka N, Desai SS, Arciero E, et al. Contemporary Review: An Overview of the Utility of Patient-Reported Outcome Measurement Information System (PROMIS) in Foot and Ankle Surgery. Foot Ankle Int 2023. https://doi.org/10.1177/10711007 231165752. 10711007231165752.

10. Usuelli FG, de Girolamo L, Grassi M, et al. All-Arthroscopic Autologous Matrix-Induced Chondrogenesis for the Treatment of Osteochondral Lesions of the Talus. Arthrosc Tech 2015;4(3):e255–9.

11. Usuelli FG, D'Ambrosi R, Maccario C, et al. All-arthroscopic AMIC® (AT-AMIC®) technique with autologous bone graft for talar osteochondral defects: clinical and radiological results. Knee Surg Sports Traumatol Arthrosc 2018;26(3):875–81.

12. Migliorini F, Eschweiler J, Maffulli N, et al. Autologous Matrix Induced Chondrogenesis (AMIC) Compared to Microfractures for Chondral Defects of the Talar Shoulder: A Five-Year Follow-Up Prospective Cohort Study. Life 2021;11(3):244.

13. McGoldrick NP, Murphy EP, Kearns SR. Osteochondral lesions of the ankle: The current evidence supporting scaffold-based techniques and biological adjuncts. Foot Ankle Surg 2018;24(2):86–91.

14. Yontar NS, Aslan L, Öğüt T. Functional Outcomes of Autologous Matrix-Related Chondrogenesis to Treat Large Osteochondral Lesions of the Talus. Foot Ankle Int 2022;43(6):783–9.

15. Ayyaswamy B, Salim M, Sidaginamale R, et al. Early to medium term outcomes of osteochondral lesions of the talus treated by autologous matrix induced chondrogenesis (AMIC). Foot Ankle Surg 2021;27(2):207–12.

16. Kubosch EJ, Erdle B, Izadpanah K, et al. Clinical outcome and T2 assessment following autologous matrix-induced chondrogenesis in osteochondral lesions of the talus. Int Orthop 2016;40(1):65–71.

17. Lee YH, Suzer F, Thermann H. Autologous Matrix-Induced Chondrogenesis in the Knee: A Review. Cartilage 2014;5(3):145–53.

18. D'Ambrosi R, Maccario C, Serra N, et al. Osteochondral Lesions of the Talus and Autologous Matrix-Induced Chondrogenesis: Is Age a Negative Predictor Outcome? Arthroscopy 2017;33(2):428–35.

19. BERNDT AL, HARTY M. Transchondral fractures (osteochondritis dissecans) of the talus. J Bone Joint Surg Am 1959;41-A:988–1020.

20. D'Ambrosi R, Maccario C, Ursino C, et al. Combining Microfractures, Autologous Bone Graft, and Autologous Matrix-Induced Chondrogenesis for the Treatment of Juvenile Osteochondral Talar Lesions. Foot Ankle Int 2017;38(5):485–95.

21. Walther M, Valderrabano V, Wiewiorski M, et al. Is there clinical evidence to support autologous matrix-induced chondrogenesis (AMIC) for chondral defects in the talus? A systematic review and meta-analysis. Foot Ankle Surg 2021;27(3):236–45.

22. D'Ambrosi R, Villafañe JH, Indino C, et al. Return to Sport After Arthroscopic Autologous Matrix-Induced Chondrogenesis for Patients With Osteochondral Lesion of the Talus. Clin J Sport Med 2019;29(6):470–5.

23. Migliorini F, Maffulli N, Baroncini A, et al. Matrix-induced autologous chondrocyte implantation versus autologous matrix-induced chondrogenesis for chondral defects of the talus: a systematic review. Br Med Bull 2021;138(1):144–54.

24. D'Ambrosi R, Maccario C, Serra N, et al. Relationship between symptomatic osteochondral lesions of the talus and quality of life, body mass index, age, size and anatomic location. Foot Ankle Surg 2018;24(4):365–72.

25. Usuelli FG, Maccario C, Ursino C, et al. The Impact of Weight on Arthroscopic Osteochondral Talar Reconstruction. Foot Ankle Int 2017;38(6):612–20.

26. Usuelli FG, Grassi M, Manzi L, et al. Treatment of osteochondral lesions of the talus with autologous collagen-induced chondrogenesis: clinical and magnetic resonance evaluation at one-year follow-up. Joints 2016;4(2):80–6.

27. Migliorini F, Schenker H, Maffulli N, et al. Autologous matrix induced chondrogenesis (AMIC) as revision procedure for failed AMIC in recurrent symptomatic osteochondral defects of the talus. Sci Rep 2022;12(1):16244.

28. Körner D, Ateschrang A, Schröter S, et al. Concomitant ankle instability has a negative impact on the quality of life in patients with osteochondral lesions of the talus: data from the German Cartilage Registry (KnorpelRegister DGOU). Knee Surg Sports Traumatol Arthrosc 2020;28(10):3339–46.

29. Richter M, Zech S, Meissner S, et al. Autologous matrix induced chondrogenesis plus peripheral blood concentrate (AMIC+PBC) in chondral lesions at the ankle as part of a complex surgical approach - 5-year follow-up. Foot Ankle Surg 2022;28(8):1321–6.

30. Shimozono Y, Brown AJ, Batista JP, et al. International Consensus Group on Cartilage Repair of the Ankle. Subchondral Pathology: Proceedings of the International Consensus Meeting on Cartilage Repair of the Ankle. Foot Ankle Int 2018;39(1_suppl):48S–53S [Erratum in: Foot Ankle Int. 2021 Feb;42(2):248].

31. D'Ambrosi R, Maccario C, Ursino C, et al. The role of bone marrow edema on osteochondral lesions of the talus. Foot Ankle Surg 2018;24(3):229–35.

32. Migliorini F, Maffulli N, Bell A, et al. Autologous Matrix-Induced Chondrogenesis (AMIC) for Osteochondral Defects of the Talus: A Systematic Review. Life 2022;12(11):1738.

33. Hollander JJ, Dahmen J, Emanuel KS, et al. The Frequency and Severity of Complications in Surgical Treatment of Osteochondral Lesions of the Talus: A Systematic Review and Meta-Analysis of 6,962 Lesions. Cartilage 2023. https://doi.org/10.1177/19476035231154746. 19476035231154746.

34. Becher C, Malahias MA, Ali MM, et al. Arthroscopic microfracture vs. arthroscopic autologous matrix-induced chondrogenesis for the treatment of articular cartilage defects of the talus. Knee Surg Sports Traumatol Arthrosc 2019;27(9): 2731–6.

35. Choi WJ, Park KK, Kim BS, et al. Osteochondral lesion of the talus: is there a critical defect size for poor outcome? Am J Sports Med 2009;37(10):1974–80.

36. Cuttica DJ, Smith WB, Hyer CF, et al. Osteochondral lesions of the talus: predictors of clinical outcome. Foot Ankle Int 2011;32(11):1045–51.

37. Gottschalk O, Altenberger S, Baumbach S, et al. Functional Medium-Term Results After Autologous Matrix-Induced Chondrogenesis for Osteochondral Lesions of the Talus: A 5-Year Prospective Cohort Study. J Foot Ankle Surg 2017;56(5):930–6.

38. Weigelt L, Hartmann R, Pfirrmann C, et al. Autologous Matrix-Induced Chondrogenesis for Osteochondral Lesions of the Talus: A Clinical and Radiological 2- to 8-Year Follow-up Study. Am J Sports Med 2019;47(7):1679–86.

39. Usuelli FG, D'Ambrosi R, Maccario C, et al. Adipose-derived stem cells in orthopaedic pathologies. Br Med Bull 2017;124(1):31–54.

40. D'Ambrosi R, Indino C, Maccario C, et al. Autologous Microfractured and Purified Adipose Tissue for Arthroscopic Management of Osteochondral Lesions of the Talus. J Vis Exp 2018;(131):56395.

41. Dombrowski ME, Yasui Y, Murawski CD, et al. International Consensus Group on Cartilage Repair of the Ankle. Conservative Management and Biological Treatment Strategies: Proceedings of the International Consensus Meeting on Cartilage Repair of the Ankle. Foot Ankle Int 2018;39(1_suppl):9S–15S [Erratum in: Foot Ankle Int. 2021 Feb;42(2):248. Erratum in: Foot Ankle Int. 2022;43(1):NP3].

42. Richter M, Zech S, Andreas Meissner S. Matrix-associated stem cell transplantation (MAST) in chondral defects of the ankle is safe and effective - 2-year-followup in 130 patients. Foot Ankle Surg 2017;23(4):236–42.

43. Roth KE, Ossendorff R, Klos K, et al. Arthroscopic Minced Cartilage Implantation for Chondral Lesions at the Talus: A Technical Note. Arthrosc Tech 2021;10(4): e1149–54.

Personalized Resurfacing for Osteochondral Lesions of the Talus

Federico Giuseppe Usuelli, MD[a], Ben Efrima, MD[a],*,
Niek Van Dijk, MD[b,c,d,e]

KEYWORDS

- Osteochondral lesion • Talus lesion • Metal inlay • Epic surf • Talus resurfacing

KEY POINTS

- Symptomatic osteochondral lesions (OLTs) of the talus are challenging to treat. Each of the available biological surgical treatment options has its indications and contraindications.
- Prefabricated metal inlay as a treatment option for osteochondral lesions of the talus has unpredictable surgical outcome.
- Patient-specific instruments have shown to improve surgical accuracy and results.
- Customized patient-specific metal inlay is a viable treatment option for OLTs and can serve as a bridge between biologics and conventional joint arthroplasty.

INTRODUCTION

Osteochondral lesions of the talus (OLTs) are the most common cause of chronic deep ankle pain.[1–3] They are characterized by damage to the cartilaginous and subchondral bone of the talar dome. Up to 75% to 100% of the OLTs are associated with underlying trauma.[1,4] These lesions can be a significant traumatic event or recurrent microtrauma.[3,5] In recent years, advancements in imaging modalities, arthroscopic techniques, and biological-based treatment have extended the surgical indication for OLTs.[5,6] For lesions up to 107 mm^2, microfracture and bone marrow stimulation (BMS) are the treatment of choice.[7] However, the clinical results of biological treatments in more extensive lesions and the results of microfracture for secondary

Contributors: All authors who have contributed to this article have agreed on the final revised version of the article.

[a] Ankle and Foot Unit, Humanitas San Pio X Hospital, Via Francesco nava 31, Milan, Italy; [b] Department of Orthopedic Surgery, Amsterdam UMC location AMC, the Netherlands; [c] Head of Ankle Unit, FIFA Medical Centre of Excellence Ripoll-DePrado Sport Clinic Madrid, Spain; [d] Head of Ankle Unit, FIFA Medical Centre of Excellence Clínica do Dragão Porto, Portugal; [e] Casa di Cura, San Rossore, Pisa, Italy

* Corresponding author. Ankle and Foot Unit, Humanitas San Pio X Hospital, Via Francesco nava 31, Milan 20159, Italy.

E-mail address: benefrima@gmail.com

Foot Ankle Clin N Am 29 (2024) 307–319
https://doi.org/10.1016/j.fcl.2023.08.001
1083-7515/24/© 2023 Elsevier Inc. All rights reserved.

surgeries are less predictable.[7,8] Osteochondral autologous transfer surgery (OATS) has been used for such lesions, but donor site morbidity is a big drawback for such a procedure.[9–11] For that reason, a focal metallic inlay was developed as a bridge between biologics and conventional joint arthroplasty.[12] Despite promising initial results, prefabricated implants are associated with unpredictable results. This article describes a novel customized patient-specific metal inlay as a treatment option for OLTs.

Etiology

The most common etiology for osteochondral defect of the talus is trauma by an ankle sprain or ankle fracture. Some lesions are non-traumatic and find their origin in ischemia, necrosis, genetics, and other idiopathic etiologies.

Raiken and colleagues used a 9-quadrant grid as a reference point to locate the OLTs; in their cohort, the medial side lesions were more predominant than the central and lateral lesions, with most medial OLT injuries located near the equation of the talar joint. The lateral injuries were found at the anterior quadrant of the talar dome (**Fig. 1**).[13,14]

The anterolateral defects are usually oval-shaped and shallow and are usually caused by an ankle sprain. The ankle rotates inside the mortise, causing a sheer force that separates the chondral, subchondral, or osteochondral layers. In contrast, the medial defects are usually deep and cup-shaped and are caused by torsional force and axial loading. The fragments can remain partially or wholly attached, while others can be displaced and become loose bodies in the joint.

Both anatomic and mechanical reasons contribute to the talus predisposition for OLTs development. The talar bone is covered with over 60% of its surface with cartilage tissue. Therefore, it has a relatively low blood supply and many watershed areas.

The ankle morphology has 2 important biomechanical characteristics that contribute to the tendency for OLTs in the face of trauma: the ankle congruency and the relatively small load-bearing area-to-forces conducted ratio. The talar dome's average cartilage thickness is 1.2 mm. In contrast, the average thickness of the hip and knee is 1.6 mm and 2.2 mm, respectively, making the ankle cartilage the thinnest with respect to the other joints in the lower limb. Shepherd and Seedhom hypothesized that the compressive loads are spread evenly across the articular surfaces in congruent joint surfaces. Therefore, the need for thick cartilage that can withstand deformities diminishes.

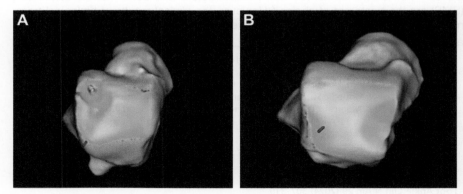

Fig. 1. (*A*) Distance map of the talar dome demonstrates an anterolateral lesion. (*B*) Distance map of the talar dome demonstrates a center medial lesion.

In contrast, incongruent joint cartilage requires withstanding deformities and is consequently covered by a thicker cartilage layer. It is hypothesized that thin cartilage has inferior shock-absorbing capabilities and reduced elasticity, rendering it susceptible to lesions.[2,3]

An important factor is the ankle's relatively low articular surface-to-force conducted ratio. Two main components are responsible for ankle shock-absorbing capabilities, the cartilage and the underlying bone. When the total cartilaginous surface diminishes due to local cartilage defect, it is associated with a load redistributing to the remaining cartilage, requiring adaptation of the joint.

Ankle trauma can affect different parts of the cartilage. A crack or fracture in the subchondral bone plate can create a gateway for joint fluid to the underlying chondral and subchondral layers. During the walking cycle, an intermittent fluid flow is pushed through this crack, reducing or inhibiting the healing of the lesions. In some cases, the remaining cartilage could act as a valve that allows liquids to flow to the subchondral layer and prevents its return. In those cases, the intraosseous pressure increases causing bone absorption and potentially cyst formation. In addition, a decrease in congruency, joint displacement, or malalignment further increases the contact pressure per cartilage area, accelerating the damage progression even further.

The clinical presentation of osteochondritis dissecans (OCD) varies between acute and chronic injury. In the acute setting, the associated injuries mask the acute cartilage injuries. The patient usually presents with swelling, limited range of motion, and pain. The injury could be associated with ankle locking if cartilage fragments displacement exists. These symptoms usually subside after 4 to 6 weeks. Chronic OLTs injuries usually manifest with deep ankle pain with a full ankle range of motion and are usually deprived of ankle swelling. Several factors play a role in pain in OLT injury: increased intraosseous pressure secondary to bone marrow edema or growing cyst volume, increased intraarticular hydrostatic pressure, and interosseous nerve-ending involvement.

Treatment

In the last decades, advancements in imaging modalities and surgical techniques have notably improved the surgical outcome for OLTs treatment. Consequently, conservative treatment for progressive and symptomatic OLTs is no longer recommended. If fragment fixation is impossible, most surgical treatments for primary OLTs are joint preserving and rely on biological treatment. Biological treatment for chondral lesions can be divided into 3 groups, bone-stimulating surgeries, osteochondral grafting, and cell-based technique.

The consensus is that for primary lesions up to 107 mm^2, microfracture and bone marrow stimulation (BMS) are the treatment of choice. However, the consensus between surgeons needs to improve regarding the optimal treatment for more extensive lesions and revision surgeries.

Guelfi and colleagues[15] evaluated the treatment algorithm for OLT of the talus across 1804 foot and ankle surgeons from different nationalities. They found a large variety of OLT management protocols across the responders. More than half of the surgeons advocated 3 months of conservative treatment, including activity restriction and physiotherapy (ranging from 4 weeks to 6 months), before proceeding to a surgical solution. The type of treatment was determined mainly by the patient's activity and demand, lesion size, presence of loose bodies, patient's age, and concomitant ankle instabilities. A total of 92% of the surgeons advocated addressing the lesion and the concomitated injuries contemporaneously, not only the lesion. Regarding the lesion size, most surgeons agree that a lesion under 15 mm should be treated only with

BMS (78%) or with additional procedures such as a scaffold or intra-articular injections (11%). In contrast, non–specific surgical tendencies were found among the participants for more extensive and deeper OLTs, reaffirming the considerable disagreement regarding the optimal biological treatments.

The second treatment option for OLTs is partial or total joint-sacrificing surgeries, such as metal resurfacing, total ankle resurfacing, and arthrodesis. These surgeries are mostly preserved for second-line treatment in middle-aged patients with extensive OLTs.

Biologic Treatments

Bone marrow–stimulating techniques

BMS surgical techniques are based on the violation of the subchondral layer. They require a debriding of the OCD, after which additional micro-fracturing or antegrade drilling can be performed. The microfracture establishes subchondral bone openings. Additionally, it disrupts intraosseous vessels. The damage to the bone and blood vessels introduces blood and bone marrow cells into the OLTs and allows a clot of scar tissue to form.[5] They are followed by fibrocartilaginous tissue replacement of the defect. BMS surgical techniques are relatively non-demanding. Recent studies indicate that BMSs are highly effective in lesions with diameters inferior to 10 mm if patients are younger than 40 years old.[16–18] However, in larger lesion diameters, older patients, and revision surgeries, BMS surgical outcome is related to less favorable results.

Some authors suggest using BMS surgery with the autologous matrix-induced chondrogenesis (AMIC) technique. During this procedure, after the standard BMSs steps, the surgeon covers the lesion site with a collagen I/III membrane that lodges the clot in place and allows for better fibrocartilage formation.[8,19,20] A meta-analysis by Walther and colleagues that included 492 patients found a statistically significant improvement in patient-reported outcomes at the 5-year follow-up. In 2015, Usuelli and colleagues[21,22] introduced an all-arthroscopic AMIC surgical technique that has reduced the need for malleolar osteotomy. AMIC is effective in lesions larger than 1 mm; however, a negative correlation between age and surgical outcome was observed. In addition, patients with a high body mass index (BMI) had less favorable outcomes.[20]

Therefore, BMS alone could be used in the minor lesion in a younger population; in a more extensive lesion, and in age-appropriate patients, BMS in conjunction with AMIC could be used. However, alternative surgical treatment should be considered in revision surgery, OLTs with a significant bone defect or bone cyst, and middle-aged patients.

Osteochondral Grafting (OG)

Osteochondral grafting is a viable treatment option for large OLTs. Currently, 2 main types of OG exist, autograft (osteochondral autologous transfer surgery [OATS] and mosaicplasty)[11,23] or fresh allograft.

Several studies have demonstrated the possible use of autologous allograft for large OLT lesions; in a meta-analysis by Feeney[11] that included 797 patients with an autologous allograft for large OLT, they found a significant improvement in both Visual Analog Scale (VAS) and American Orthopedic Foot and Ankle Score (AOFAS) scores with a mean follow-up of 47.7 months. A meta-analysis by Seow and colleagues[24] evaluated 205 ankles of athletic patients treated with autograft. They found that 86.3% of the patients returned to play, and 81.8% reported returning to preinjury status. A significant side effect is donor site morbidity. For knee-to-ankle transplants, the average donor-side morbidity is 19.6%. And when considering centers that only do a limited number of these OATS procedures(less the 20 procedures), the donor side morbidity is even 37%[25]

Another grafting technique involves the use of fresh allograft. This surgical technique has a few advantages since it does not require graft harvesting from an asymptomatic surgical site and could be fitted precisely to a particular surgical site. A systemic review by Pereira and colleagues[26] evaluated 191 patients treated with fresh allograft for OLT of the talus. They found a significant improvement in AOFAS and VAS scores and an overall graft survivor rate of 86.6%.

The benefit of both techniques stems from the ability to provide hyaluronic cartilage and structural bone support. In contrast, BMS techniques do not provide structural bone support, producing fibrocartilage tissue with inferior qualities concerning hyaluronic cartilage. Jerkin and colleagues compared the clinical results between patients under and over 40 years old and found satisfactory results in the patient-reported outcome and graft survival in both age groups.[18] However, these techniques have limitations. The autograft technique is associated with 9% to 15% of donor site morbidity.[23,27] Whereas frozen allograft and fresh frozen allograft had an unacceptable failure rate; therefore, only the more expensive and less available option, fresh allografts, are used. In addition, this technique carries an increased risk of disease transmission.[26]

OG surgeries are often associated with graft failure, cyst development, and progressive osteoarthritis. Moreover, both techniques are time-consuming and require advanced surgical skills. Finally, achieving anatomic congruence, graft incorporation, and complete healing can be difficult.[27]

Cell-based therapy

BMS techniques rely on the induction of fibrocartilage regeneration. In contrast, the principle behind cell-based treatment approaches is the ability of transplanted chondrocytes to generate a hyaline-like repair tissue with biochemical and biomechanical properties closer to the native articular tissue. Autologous chondrocyte implantation (ACI)[5] is a 2-stage procedure in which chondrocytes are harvested during the initial procedure, expanded in culture, and then reimplanted to the defect in a second procedure. Matrix-associated chondrocyte implantation [5] involves culturing the harvested chondrocytes on collagen or hyaluronic acid–base matrices before implantation. Using this technique, a more even spread to the chondrocytes is obtained. In a large meta-analysis, Mu Hu et al[23] reported that 458 patients reported an 89% success rate and 86.3% improvement in patient-reported outcomes. A vital shortcoming of this technique is that it is not readily available since it requires an advanced lab to cultivate the cells. They do not provide structural support in cases of a significant bone defect.

Metal implants

The notion of using partial or total metal resurfacing has existed for a while. Sir Jhon Charnley introduced it to orthopedic surgery in the 1960s. Partial and complete resurfacing has been widely accepted in hip and shoulder surgery. However, only in recent years has joint resurfacing been reintroduced for knee and ankle surgery. The main goal of this surgical technique is to recreate the ankle anatomy based on intraoperative topographic mapping.

This technique also allows concomitant soft tissue and bony surgical procedures since the metal components do not increase joint volume. The additional benefit is that metal resurfacing is performed with limited surgical exposure, reduced surgical time, simple surgical technique, and scarce blood loss. The success of the resurfacing is based on the implant integration into the surrounding bone, the integrity of the surrounding cartilage, the adherence of the healthy cartilage of the implants, and a correct redistribution of the joint load on the surrounding cartilage.

The main indications are symptomatic middle-aged (35–60 years)[18] active patients with an osteochondral defect of greater than107 mm[27] with significant subchondral bone defects (subchondral cysts) and a history of failed first-line biological treatments. This method can be regarded as the final attempt at joint preservation surgery in a symptomatic young patient before continuing to the joint sacrificing procedure.

Over the last decade, Hemicap,[28–30] a prefabricated focal prosthetic inlay adapted from knee surgery, was introduced as a second-line salvage treatment for OLTs. The initial results were encouraging. Vuurberg et al[29] analyzed 38 patients treated with Hemicap. The study's mean follow-up time was 5.1 years. They reported improved patient-reported outcomes and good patient satisfaction with only 2 revision cases. Other case series demonstrate less favorable results. Ettinger and colleagues[31] reported a 50% revision rate and pointed out that patients with increased BMI treated with Hemicap have a poor prognosis. Maiorano et al[28], in a different study, reported unsatisfactory pain improvement. A few authors have raised concerns about the implant that could explain the outcome discrepancy. First, this implant had only 15 offset configurations, and since there is wide variability in talus morphology,[32] it is highly challenging to reconstruct the complex morphology of the talar dome. An additional limitation of this system is implanting positioning; a biomechanical study highlighted that metal resurfacing could recover more than 90% of the contact area. However, if the implant protrudes by 0.25 mm, peak contact stress increases by 220%. In case the implant recessed 0.25 mm, the peak values of implant-on-cartilage contact stress decreased, while there was an increase in peak values of the cartilage-on-cartilage contact area.[30] Therefore, the surgical results are influenced by the surgeon's ability to position the component in the correct location and depth.

Patient-specific instruments

During the last decade, a few groundbreaking technologies were introduced to foot and ankle surgery. This technology allows tailoring a patient-specific surgery that considers each patient's unique anatomy. Advanced imaging techniques currently enable surgeons to create individualized preoperative plans. Using this plan, surgeons can manufacture patient-specific "tool kits" with customized operative guides and implants. In ankle arthroplasties, weight-bearing computed tomography for preoperative plans and customized implants have been proven to improve surgical accuracy in many studies.[33] Premanufactured focal implants for osteochondral currently demonstrate limited ability and are technically demanding. In order not to compromise on implant location, size, and shape,novel patient-specific metallic inlay for OLTs and focal cartilage defect of the knee was proposed. The currently available literature is scarce. Stålman and colleagues [34] used customized femoral condyle implants for focal cartilage injuries. In a short-term study, they reported no implant migration and good subjective outcomes at the 12-month follow-up. Al-Bayati et al.[35] evaluated the surgical outcome of customized knee metal inlay at the 5-year follow-up. They reconfirmed that improvement persisted, there was no conversion to total knee replacement, and only 1 patient had progression in OA changes. Specifically, in OLTs treatment, a case report by Holtz et al[36] evaluated the result of a 33-year-old physically active patient with a history of large OLTs in the medial aspect of the talar dome. After a failed conservative and AOTS treatment, he was treated with patient-specific metallic inlay (Episealer Talus Implant, Episurf Medical, Stockholm, Sweden).

At the 5-year follow-up, he reported subjective improvement and a total return to a highly demanding sports activity. The promising results of patient-specific instruments metal inlay for a focal osteochondral lesion in the knee and talus are encouraging. Furthermore, it indicates that it could become a valuable bridging treatment.

Indication and Contraindications

Indication criteria

1. Focal medial or lateral OLTs of the talar dome.
2. Lesion osteochondral lesion of greater than or equal to 12 mm, (>107 mm^2).
3. Symptomatic OLTs causing deep ankle pain unresponsive to conventional conservative treatments.
4. Age between 18 and 65 years.
5. BMI less than35.
6. Absence of joint space narrowing in standard radiographs. (Osteophytes are not considered a contraindication).

Absolute contraindications

1. Non-focal defects demonstrated on an MRI scan.
2. Ongoing infection in the ankle joint.
3. Inflammatory arthritis or radiographic osteoarthritis in the ankle joint.
4. Sensitivity to cobalt–chrome alloys and materials typically used in prosthetic devices.
5. Inadequate bone stock where the Episealer is to be inserted.
6. Existing prosthesis in the area of treatment or opposing surface.
7. Severe lesion on the opposing tibial surface.

Relative contraindications include

1. Pain of unknown etiology
2. Demineralized bone
3. Instability or malalignment in the ankle joint (maximum 5° malalignment)
4. Other diseases or medications that may affect the bone anchoring of the Episealer
5. An uncooperative patient that is not willing to follow instructions.
6. Muscular insufficiency
7. Vascular insufficiency
8. Medical, hormonal, hematological, immunologic, or metabolic illnesses

Image analysis and implant design

Based on a preoperative MRI, a patient-specific virtual 3-dimensional (3D) model of the focal osteochondral lesion is created digitally and used to design an individualized metal implant and corresponding instruments before the surgery (**Fig. 2**). During the damage mapping (Damage Marking Report), the cartilage and bone structure of the talar dome and the tibial plafond are assessed. The assessment must confirm localized isolated cartilage damage in the talar dome without an opposing cartilage defect or other comorbidities. Based on the 3D joint model, an implant is designed to cover the entire defect of cartilage and underlying bone.

The metal implant is a cobalt–chrome alloy covered with titanium (undercoating) and hydroxyapatite (outer coating). Both joint-facing layers have a thickness of approximately 60 μm and are in the center of the implant. The implant has 1 or 2 centered pins to ensure immediate fixation. The Episealer is manufactured on a custom-made basis.

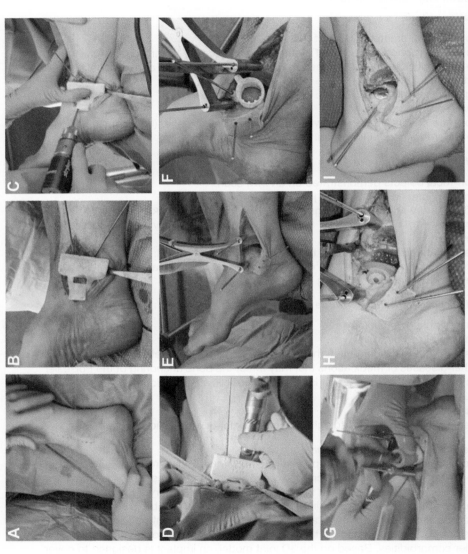

Fig. 2. Episurf surgical technique is performed using a medial approach to the ankle (*A*). A patient-specific osteotomy guide is placed over the medial malleolus and secured using 2 K-wire (*B*). Initially, 2 holes are drilled to prepare the malleolus for fixation at the end of the surgery (*C*). After that, an osteotomy is performed (*D*). The medial malleolus is removed, and the OLT is exposed (*E*). The guide is placed over the OLT (*F*). Through the epiguide,

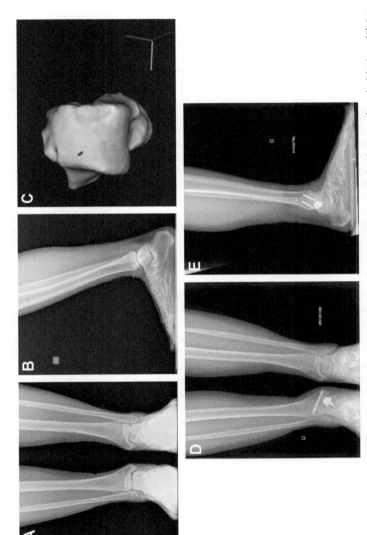

Fig. 3. (A) Preoperative weight-bearing X-rays in an anteroposterior (AP) view showing a medial side osteochondral lesion. (B) Preoperative weight-bearing X-rays in lateral view showing an osteochondral lesion. (C) Preoperative weight-bearing computed tomography (CT) showing medial osteochondral lesion. (D) Sixteen months postoperative weight-bearing X-ray in an AP view showing an Episurf metal implant. (E) Postoperative 16-month follow-up weight-bearing X rays in lateral view showing an Episurf implant.

Surgical Technique

In order to access the articular surface for a medial lesion, an osteotomy of the medial malleolus is required. The surgery is conducted in the supine position. A tourniquet usage is recommended. The surgery can be performed with general or spinal anesthesia. For the osteotomy, a patient-specific osteotomy guide is placed. This ensures the correct location and depth of the osteotomy. The guide also contains 2 drill holes for the screws used to fix the osteotomy at the end of the procedure. After the osteotomy and posterior capsular release, the malleolus is displaced. A bone spreader facilitates the placement of the Epiguide. This patient-specific drill polyamide guide (Epiguide) produced by a 3D printer is placed and secured with 2 K-wires on the bone surrounding the defect. Through the Epiguide, the defect is drilled. The drill has a deep stop to prevent over-reaming and can be adjusted by 0.2 mm steps. The implant is delivered with a 3D-printed dummy (Epidummy) that simulates the implant. The dummy ensures that the drilling is deep enough and that the Episealer is not protruding and implanted at the "save zone" 0.4 mm below the native cartilage surface. A dummy is positioned to check if the depth is correct. If the resection is deep enough, the implant can be inserted. Implanting the component 0.4 to 0.6 mm under the adjacent cartilage border is essential to avoid damage to the opposite tibial cartilage. The tibia-oriented surface of the implant (diameter 15 mm) is designed to mimic the talus's original curvature. After implantation, the osteotomized tibia is reduced and fixated with 2 screws. The capsular and subcutaneous tissue and the skin are closed after lavage. Postoperative care includes 6 weeks of partial weight bearing with crutches until the osteotomy consolidated.

THE AUTHOR'S OPINION

Treating symptomatic OLTs can be challenging, especially since the current literature lacks a clear consensus on how to treat extensive lesions, revision cases, and the older population. Emerging technologies offer an opportunity to enable tailor-made patient-specific treatment solutions. Introducing a new surgical technique or technology should follow a specific, stepwise validation process, including concept/theory formation, procedure development and exploration, procedure assessment, and long-term evidence-based studies.[37] The authors have a positive experience with custom-made metal inlays for OLTs (**Fig. 3**). However, long-term follow-up and larger cohorts are required. The authors believe that this technique is proven effective. The authors expect that the indications for metal inlays as a solution for focal osteochondral talar defect will broaden toward other indications, such as primary focal defects.

CLINICS CARE POINTS

- Preoperative evaluation should include careful assessment of the lower limb alignment and concomitant injuries.
- Any concomitant injuries should be addressed during the OLT surgeries.
- A preoperative evaluation must include an assessment of the OLT dimension, depth, and location.
- The surgeon should tailor a surgical treatment that fits the lesions' morphology.
- Symptomatic Lesions with a diameter inferior to 107 mm could be treated with microfracture. Microfracture shows a less predictable outcome and requires other surgical solutions.

- Preoperative planning using 3D modeling and patient-specific instruments improves surgical accuracy.
- Personalized resurfacing for osteochondral lesions of the talus could serve as a bridging treatment in OLT with significant bone defects and revision surgery.

CONFLICT OF INTEREST

F.G. Usuelli: consultant for ZimmerBiomeet, Episurf, Artrex, Paragon, Gelistlich, planmed. International editor for Foot and Ankle international. N. Van Dijk: consultant for Episurf and Editor ibn chief for Journal of ISAKOS.

REFERENCES

1. Bruns J, Habermann C, Werner M. Osteochondral Lesions of the Talus: A Review on Talus Osteochondral Injuries, Including Osteochondritis Dissecans. Cartilage 2021;13(1_suppl):1380s–401s.
2. van Dijk CN, Reilingh ML, Zengerink M, et al. Osteochondral defects in the ankle: why painful? Knee Surg Sports Traumatol Arthrosc 2010;18(5):570–80.
3. van Dijk CN, Reilingh ML, Zengerink M, et al. The natural history of osteochondral lesions in the ankle. Instr Course Lect 2010;59:375–86.
4. Rikken QGH, Kerkhoffs G. Osteochondral Lesions of the Talus: An Individualized Treatment Paradigm from the Amsterdam Perspective. Foot Ankle Clin 2021; 26(1):121–36.
5. Zengerink M, Struijs PA, Tol JL, et al. Treatment of osteochondral lesions of the talus: a systematic review. Knee Surg Sports Traumatol Arthrosc 2010;18(2):238–46.
6. Verhagen RA, Struijs PA, Bossuyt PM, et al. Systematic review of treatment strategies for osteochondral defects of the talar dome. Foot Ankle Clin 2003;8(2): 233–42, viii-ix.
7. Ramponi L, Yasui Y, Murawski CD, et al. Lesion Size Is a Predictor of Clinical Outcomes After Bone Marrow Stimulation for Osteochondral Lesions of the Talus: A Systematic Review. Am J Sports Med 2017;45(7):1698–705.
8. Migliorini F, Maffulli N, Bell A, et al. Autologous Matrix-Induced Chondrogenesis (AMIC) for Osteochondral Defects of the Talus: A Systematic Review. Life 2022; 12(11). https://doi.org/10.3390/life12111738.
9. Dahmen J, Lambers KTA, Reilingh ML, et al. No superior treatment for primary osteochondral defects of the talus. Knee Surg Sports Traumatol Arthrosc 2018; 26(7):2142–57.
10. Hunt KJ, Ebben BJ. Management of Treatment Failures in Osteochondral Lesions of the Talus. Foot Ankle Clin 2022;27(2):385–99.
11. Feeney KM. The Effectiveness of Osteochondral Autograft Transfer in the Management of Osteochondral Lesions of the Talus: A Systematic Review and Meta-Analysis. Cureus. Nov 2022;14(11):e31337.
12. van Bergen CJ, van Eekeren IC, Reilingh ML, et al. Treatment of osteochondral defects of the talus with a metal resurfacing inlay implant after failed previous surgery: a prospective study. Bone Joint Lett J 2013;95-b(12):1650–5.
13. van Diepen PR, Dahmen J, Altink JN, et al. Location Distribution of 2,087 Osteochondral Lesions of the Talus. Cartilage 2021;13(1_suppl):1344s–53s.
14. Elias I, Zoga AC, Morrison WB, et al. Osteochondral lesions of the talus: localization and morphologic data from 424 patients using a novel anatomical grid scheme. Foot Ankle Int 2007;28(2):154–61.

15. Guelfi M, DiGiovanni CW, Calder J, et al. Large variation in management of talar osteochondral lesions among foot and ankle surgeons: results from an international survey. Knee Surg Sports Traumatol Arthrosc 2021;29(5):1593–603.

16. Rikken QGH, Dahmen J, Stufkens SAS, et al. Satisfactory long-term clinical outcomes after bone marrow stimulation of osteochondral lesions of the talus. Knee Surg Sports Traumatol Arthrosc 2021;29(11):3525–33.

17. Powers RT, Dowd TC, Giza E. Surgical Treatment for Osteochondral Lesions of the Talus. Arthroscopy 2021;37(12):3393–6.

18. Jeuken RM, van Hugten PPW, Roth AK, et al. A Systematic Review of Focal Cartilage Defect Treatments in Middle-Aged Versus Younger Patients. Orthop J Sports Med 2021;9(10). https://doi.org/10.1177/23259671211031244. 23259671211031244.

19. Walther M, Valderrabano V, Wiewiorski M, et al. Is there clinical evidence to support autologous matrix-induced chondrogenesis (AMIC) for chondral defects in the talus? A systematic review and meta-analysis. Foot Ankle Surg 2021;27(3):236–45.

20. Jantzen C, Ebskov LB, Johansen JK. AMIC Procedure for Treatment of Osteochondral Lesions of Talus-A Systematic Review of the Current Literature. J Foot Ankle Surg 2022;61(4):888–95.

21. Usuelli FG, de Girolamo L, Grassi M, et al. All-Arthroscopic Autologous Matrix-Induced Chondrogenesis for the Treatment of Osteochondral Lesions of the Talus. Arthrosc Tech 2015;4(3):e255–9.

22. D'Ambrosi R, Villafañe JH, Indino C, et al. Return to Sport After Arthroscopic Autologous Matrix-Induced Chondrogenesis for Patients With Osteochondral Lesion of the Talus. Clin J Sport Med 2019;29(6):470–5.

23. Hu M, Li X, Xu X. Efficacy and safety of autologous chondrocyte implantation for osteochondral defects of the talus: a systematic review and meta-analysis. Arch Orthop Trauma Surg 2023;143(1):71–9.

24. Seow D, Shimozono Y, Gianakos AL, et al. Autologous osteochondral transplantation for osteochondral lesions of the talus: high rate of return to play in the athletic population. Knee Surg Sports Traumatol Arthrosc 2021;29(5):1554–61.

25. Andrade R, Vasta S, Pereira R, et al. Knee donor-site morbidity after mosaicplasty - a systematic review. J Exp Orthop 2016;3(1):31.

26. Pereira GF, Steele JR, Fletcher AN, et al. Fresh Osteochondral Allograft Transplantation for Osteochondral Lesions of the Talus: A Systematic Review. J Foot Ankle Surg May-Jun 2021;60(3):585–91.

27. Anwander H, Vetter P, Kurze C, et al. Evidence for operative treatment of talar osteochondral lesions: a systematic review. EFORT Open Rev 2022;7(7):460–9.

28. Maiorano E, Bianchi A, Hosseinzadeh MK, et al. HemiCAP® implantation after failed previous surgery for osteochondral lesions of the talus. Foot Ankle Surg 2021;27(1):77–81.

29. Vuurberg G, Reilingh ML, van Bergen CJA, et al. Metal Resurfacing Inlay Implant for Osteochondral Talar Defects After Failed Previous Surgery: A Midterm Prospective Follow-up Study. Am J Sports Med 2018;46(7):1685–92.

30. van Bergen CJ, Zengerink M, Blankevoort L, et al. Novel metallic implantation technique for osteochondral defects of the medial talar dome. A cadaver study. Acta Orthop 2010;81(4):495–502.

31. Ettinger S, Stukenborg-Colsman C, Waizy H, et al. Results of HemiCAP(®) Implantation as a Salvage Procedure for Osteochondral Lesions of the Talus. J Foot Ankle Surg 2017;56(4):788–92.

32. D'Ambrosi R, Usuelli FG. Osteochondral lesions of the talus: are we ready for metal? Ann Transl Med 2018;6(Suppl 1):S19.

33. Zeitlin J, Henry J, Ellis S. Preoperative Guidance With Weight-Bearing Computed Tomography and Patient-Specific Instrumentation in Foot and Ankle Surgery. Hss j 2021;17(3):326–32.

34. Stålman A, Sköldenberg O, Martinez-Carranza N, et al. No implant migration and good subjective outcome of a novel customized femoral resurfacing metal implant for focal chondral lesions. Knee Surg Sports Traumatol Arthrosc 2018; 26(7):2196–204.

35. Al-Bayati M, Martinez-Carranza N, Roberts D, et al. Good subjective outcome and low risk of revision surgery with a novel customized metal implant for focal femoral chondral lesions at a follow-up after a minimum of 5 years. Arch Orthop Trauma Surg 2022;142(10):2887–92.

36. Holz J, Spalding T, Boutefnouchet T, et al. Patient-specific metal implants for focal chondral and osteochondral lesions in the knee; excellent clinical results at 2 years. Knee Surg Sports Traumatol Arthrosc 2021;29(9):2899–910.

37. Factor S, Khoury A, Atzmon R, et al. Combined endoscopic and mini-open repair of chronic complete proximal hamstring tendon avulsion: a novel approach and short-term outcomes. J Hip Preserv Surg 2020;7(4):721–7.

Ankle Instability
Facts and Myths to Protect Your Cartilage Repairing

Yuhan Tan, MD[a,b,*], Kristian Buedts, MD[a]

KEYWORDS

• Osteochondral lesion • Talus • Cartilage • Ankle • Instability

KEY POINTS

- Up to 80% of patients with an osteochondral lesion of the talus (OLT) reported a history of trauma. Acute trauma, as well as repetitive microtrauma associated with chronic instability, is a cause of cartilage lesions.
- We propose the "HALO" approach when dealing with patients with an OLT. The "HALO" acronym stands for patient *History*, *Alignment*, *Ligamentous* (in)stability, and *Others*. This approach can be applied in primary cases or after failed treatment of an OLT.
- Many studies investigating the outcome of OLT do not mention ankle instability. We believe that achieving a stable ankle is the key. Therefore, if present, concomitant ankle instability should be addressed. Conservative treatment may be effective, but if instability persists, surgical intervention may be necessary.
- The timing of surgery for an OLT depends on the characteristics of the OLT and any associated lesions. If associated (ligamentous) lesions require a more urgent surgical treatment, we recommend treating the OLT in the same session, and vice versa. When surgically treating ankle instability and OLT, we recommend a single-stage surgical approach.

INTRODUCTION

Ankle injuries are the most common lower limb musculoskeletal injury. Over the past 2 decades, extensive research has shown that ankle sprains cause more damage to the ankle joint than was previously thought. Of the patients experiencing an ankle sprain, 20% will eventually progress into developing chronic ankle instability (CAI).[1] Patients with CAI typically present with complaints of ankle pain, swelling, "giving-away," and a history of recurrent ankle sprains.

[a] Department of Orthopaedics, ZNA Middelheim, Lindendreef 12020 Antwerp, Belgium;
[b] Department of Orthopaedics, University Hospital Brussels, Laarbeeklaan 101, 1090 Jette, Belgium
* Corresponding author.
E-mail address: yuhantan@hotmail.com

Foot Ankle Clin N Am 29 (2024) 321–331
https://doi.org/10.1016/j.fcl.2023.07.005
1083-7515/24/© 2023 Elsevier Inc. All rights reserved.

Acute trauma and repetitive micro-traumata due to ankle instability and/or hind foot malalignment seem to be a leading cause of osteochondral lesions of the talus (OLTs).[2] Previous studies have shown that up to 80% of osteochondral injuries reported a history of trauma.[3,4] If untreated, chronic lateral ankle instability (CLAI) will eventually progress to post-traumatic ankle osteoarthritis due to pathologic stress on cartilage surfaces[5,6] Other causes of OLT include genetic, vascular, and endocrine factors.[7–9]

Non-operative treatment of OLT consists of immobilization, anti-inflammatory medication, viscosupplementation, physical therapy, and orthotics and is recommended for at least 3 months.[5] However, associated lesions can affect the timing of surgery and may require a more urgent surgical approach.[2] Unfortunately, articular cartilage has a low potential for intrinsic repair and regeneration.[10] Successful non-operative treatment of OLT has been reported in about 50% of the cases.[11] Currently, the most commonly used operative methods include fixation of the fragment with or without debridement and cancellous bone grafting[12,13]; debridement with or without bone marrow stimulation (microfracture)[14]; autologous matrix-induced chondrogenesis (AMIC)[15]; matrix-induced autologous chondrocyte transplantation (MACI)[16]; and autologous or allogenic osteo (chondral) transplantation (AOT).[17,18]

ANATOMY

The ankle (talocrular) joint is a highly congruent joint including 3 articulations: the tibiotalar, talofibular, and tibiofibular joints. The talus articulates with the tibia superiorly and medially, and with the fibula laterally. The talus is wider anteriorly, which provides stabilization in dorsiflexion.[19] The talus has no muscular attachments and is in large depended on ligamentous structures to maintain its congruence in the ankle joint. Together with the ligamentous structures, the muscles and tendons also contribute to maintain a correct position of the talus in the ankle mortise.[20]

Lateral Ligament Complex

The major lateral ligaments are the anterior talofibular ligament (ATFL), the calcaneofibular ligament (CFL), and the posterior talofibular ligament (PTFL). The ATFL typically shows a double-banded morphology and is separated by vascular branches.[21,22] It restricts internal rotation of the talus in the mortise and inversion during plantarflexion, while the PTFL is an important stabilizer especially when the ankle is in dorsiflexion[23,24] The CFL is structurally 2.5 times stronger than the ATFL and is nearly exclusively responsible for resistance to inversion during dorsiflexion in the neutral state. During plantarflexion, the CFL resists inversion alongside the ATFL and acts as a stabilizer of the subtalar joint.[24]

Medial Ligament Complex

The deltoid ligament is fan-shaped and comprises the anterior and posterior tibiotalar ligaments, the tibionavicular ligament, and the tibiocalcaneal ligament.[25] It consists of a deep and superficial portion and plays an essential role in stability against valgus and rotational forces.[26]

Syndesmosis

The syndesmosis is an essential stabilizer of the ankle joint and consists of a complex ligamentous structure with 3 different portions: the anterior inferior tibiofibular ligament (AITFL); the interosseous ligament (IOL); and the posterior inferior tibiofibular and the transverse ligaments (PITFL and TL). The posterior syndesmosis plays the most important role providing 40% to 45% of the resistance to diastasis, while the AITFL provides around 35%.[27,28]

THE ROLE OF LIGAMENTS ON CARTILAGE INTEGRITY

Both acute and chronic injury-associated changes in joint stability contribute to a pathomechanical loading environment that leads to cartilage degeneration.[29,30] One of the most widely used techniques to measure cartilage alterations is MRI T2 and T2* relaxation time mapping.[31] Elevated T2 and T2* values (expressed in milliseconds) are associated with the loss or disorganized arrangement of the collagen fibril network and increased water content, suggesting cartilage degeneration.[32,33] T2 and T2* mapping have benefits in diagnosing cartilage irregularities and in the follow-up after cartilage treatment procedures.A study investigating patients with partial and complete ATFL tears shows that more than 6 months after trauma, a significant increase in T2 value can be found in the medial anterior and lateral anterior compartments of the talus. The subjects with complete ATFL tears also had elevated T2 values in the lateral central compartment of the talus.[34] However, the relationship between T2 values and clinical outcome is unclear. Although patients exhibited improved clinical outcomes after lateral anatomic repair, the elevated T2 values did not fully recover at 3 years of follow-up.[35] This could indicate that the cartilage degeneration in patients with CAI might not be fully reversible after anatomic repair. However, it also shows that there was no further cartilage degeneration after anatomic repair.

Hunt demonstrated that sectioning of the CFL ligament in cadavers resulted in an important decrease in stiffness and peak torque in the tibiotalar joint. Also, tibiotalar mean contact area increased significantly and more inversion of the talus and calcaneum was seen with weight-bearing inversion after sectioning of the CFL.[24] Moreover, when both the ATFL and CFL were sectioned, the center of force moved medially and posteriorly, which is the most common location of osteochondral lesions of the talus.[36] Alterations in forces in the tibiotalar joint may lead to more severe cartilage damage, even when subjected to forces that would not necessarily result in injury.[24]

Clinical Evaluation

When treating OLT, one should also treat the underlying cause of the OLT. The majority of patients presenting with an OLT reported a history of trauma.[3,4] An OLT can also develop as a result of chronic overloading, as is the case in untreated instability or malalignment.[37]

To assist with the clinical evaluation, we propose the "HALO" approach. The "HALO"acronym refers to the evaluation of patient *History, Alignment, Ligamentous* (in)stability, and *Others*. This approach can be applied in primary OLT cases but should also be considered after failed treatment.

H – History. A thorough medical history is the basis of every treatment plan. Patientssuffering from an OLT usually present with deep non-specific ankle pain 6 to 12 months afteran initial trauma. It is important to question the occurrence of a previous sprain, the trauma mechanism, and complaints of CAI. Mechanical symptoms such as blocking or clicking should also be questioned.

A – Alignment. When treating any cartilage lesion, one should always look at the alignment of the affected limb. This includes the alignment of the hind foot and the whole lower limb. Uncorrected malalignment will cause eccentric loading on the ankle joint.[38] This eccentric loading may affect the ability of cartilage to heal.

L – Ligaments. One should always look for signs of instability in patients with osteochondral lesions. A thorough physical examination should be done to detect signs of lateral, medial, and syndesmotic instability. Limitations of ankle, subtalar, and talonavicular range of motion should also be examined.

O – Others: One should also look for other causes and other lesions. Other causes of OLT include vascular, endocrine, and genetic factors. Loose bodies can be present and may require an additional posterior arthroscopy (**Figs. 1** and **2**).

RADIOGRAPHIC EVALUATION

While a thorough history and physical examination are essential, a treatment plan cannot be made without additional radiologic examination. Plain radiographs can visualize OLTs but have a relatively low sensitivity, missing about 50% of cases.[39] MRI is better able to visualize ankle cartilage, underlying bone edema, and accompanying injuries to ligaments and tendons. Computed tomography (CT) provides a superior assessment of the subchondral bone and can more accurately predict the depth and size of the OLT.[40] Intra-articular contrast can help assess the stability of the OLT but is an invasive procedure.[41] A standing cone-beam CT (CBCT) has similar advantages to a CT scan and can be useful in detecting unstable syndesmotic lesions and evaluating hind foot alignment.[42,43]

TREATMENT

Many of the existing studies investigating the outcome after surgical treatment of OLTs exclude patients with ankle instability or do not mention investigating ankle instability in their cohorts. As previously noted, we believe it is important to identify any signs of concomitant ankle instability, as this should be integrated into the treatment plan. In general, treatment of OLT should be personalized based on patient factors (age, body mass index, level of activity, patients' expectations), OLT characteristics (location, size and debt, duration of symptoms, and displacement), and other relevant factors such as lower limb and hind foot alignment, ankle stability, and other concomitant injuries. Non-operative treatment of symptomatic OLT has a relatively low success rate. A systematic review by Zengerink reported a success rate of non-operative treatment in approximately 50% of the patients.[11] The relatively low success rate can be explained by the low intrinsic healing capacity of hyaline cartilage. However, other factors such as ankle instability were not investigated as a potential contributing factor.

When ankle instability is present, a treatment should be developed to regain ankle stability and reduce the risk of (micro)trauma to the articular cartilage. Ankle stability

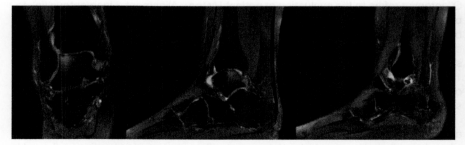

Fig. 1. A 19-year-old female patient presented with deep ankle pain and recurrent ankle sprains. She sustained her first ankle sprain during skateboarding at the age of 15 year old. MRI shows an osteochondral lesion of the lateral talar dome (*left and middle image*). Sagittal image shows a loose body in the posterior part of the ankle joint (*right image*).

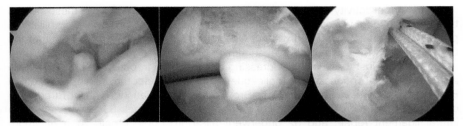

Fig. 2. Treatment of the same patient (image 1); Single-stage posterior and anterior arthroscopy was performed. Left image: posterior arthroscopy showing the cartilage loose body in the posterolateral corner. Middle image: cartilage loose body before removal. Right image: anterior arthroscopy for arthroscopic stabilization and bone marrow stimulation of the OLT. Image showing the anchor placement for arthroscopic lateral stabilization.

can be achieved through conservative or operative treatment. Conservative treatment is usually applied for 3 to 6 months and includes physiotherapy, bracing, and a gradual return to activity. If instability persists, surgical treatment is recommended. The Broström procedure, with or without modifications, is still considered the gold-standard procedure for lateral ankle instability. Other techniques include arthroscopic techniques and the use of augments.[44] In cases of inadequate ligamentous or capsular tissue or in revision surgery, a ligamentous anatomic reconstruction with an autograft or allograft is indicated.[45] Medial instability can be addressed by direct repair or reconstruction of the deltoid ligament. A higher level of awareness is required when dealing with symptomatic syndesmotic lesions. In case of unstable syndesmotic lesions or lesions not responding to conservative treatment, operative repair or reconstruction may be necessary. Debate continues on the superiority of different syndesmotic fixation techniques.

If associated (ligamentous) lesions require a more urgent surgical treatment, we recommend treating the OLT in the same session, and vice versa.

SURGICAL TREATMENT
Outcome of Stabilization Procedures

Most of the existing studies have focused on the outcome of lateral stabilization procedures with concomitant osteochondral talar lesions. Jiang and colleagues. examined the outcomes of anatomic lateral ligament repair in patients with CLAI, comparing those with and without concomitant OLTs. The study followed 70 patients who underwent anatomic lateral ligament repair (open modified Broström) and were divided into 2 groups: those with an OLT (34 out of 70) and those without an OLT (36 out of 70). Osteochondral lesions were small (15 mm^2 and < 8 mm in depth) and were treated by arthroscopic abrasion, curettage, drilling, or microfracture. At 45 months of follow-up, both groups achieved similar results regarding patient satisfaction, visual analog scale (VAS), and American Orthopedic Foot and Ankle Society (AOFAS) scores. However, the study did find that more patients in the OLT group (8/34) experienced a slight, non-significant decrease in range of motion compared to the non-OLT group (2/36).[46] Feng and colleagues retrospectively studied 90 patients with CLAI with and without medial OLT. They performed an arthroscopic Broströmprocedure in all patients and performed an additional microfracture in patients with an OLT (60 out of 90). At 24 months of follow-up, they found no statistical difference between the OLT and non-OLT group in terms of VAS, AOFAS scores, Karlsson Ankle Function scores , Anterior Talar Translation , Active Joint Position Sense , time of return to normal activity, or the rate of return to pre-injury sports.[47] While these studies by Jiang and Feng were designed to investigate the outcome of a lateral stabilization procedure in patients with and without OLT, it is also interesting to observe that the OLT patients in these studiesachieved similar outcomes to those without OLT after addressing the instability.When addressing the instability in patients with OLT, there are many surgical options.Xu and colleagues studied the outcome of an open modified Broström repair versus anarthroscopic Broström repair in patients with OLT (requiring debridement or microfracture). In their cohort of 67 patients, 35 underwent open lateral ligament repair, and 32 underwent all-arthroscopic repair. At a minimum follow-up of 24 months, both groups showed significant improvements in functional outcome scores compared to preoperative scores. There was no significant difference in patient satisfaction, VAS score (1.8 ± 1.6 vs 2.1 ± 1.7; $P = .73$),AOFAS score (87.7 ± 7.6 vs 86.9 ± 7.3; $P = .77$), Karlsson score (83.1 ± 8.2 vs81.7 ± 9.1; $P = .89$), or Tegner score (5.5 ± 2.3 vs 5.0 ± 2.1; $P = .72$) between the 2groups.[48] Treatment of chronic lateral instability and OLT can be in a single-stage or a staged surgical approach. Wei and colleagues performed single-stage surgery in 52 patients and a staged surgery in 51 patients. They performed an open modified Broström procedure for the CLAI and an arthroscopic cartilage debridement or microfracture treatment for the OLT. In the staged approach group, the lateral ligamentous stabilization procedure was performed 4 to 6 months after the OLT treatment. The authors found no inferiority in the single-stage surgery group. In fact, AOFAS scores 85 (interquartile range,76–89) versus 79.5 (70–87) and Karlsson– Peterson scores 79 (70–85) versus 75 (65–80) were significantly higher at 12 months of follow-up in the single-stage surgery group. At 24 months and at the end of follow-up (almost 60 months), there was no more difference between the 2 groups.[49]

Outcome of Osteochondral Lesion of the Talus Treatment

While several studies suggest treating ankle instability in the presence of OLT, the available evidence in the literature remains limited.[2,50,51] Currently, the most common intervention for OLT is bone marrow stimulation. A review by Rikken studied the long-term outcome of bone marrow stimulation for small OLTs in 323 ankles. They reported satisfactory patient outcomes, with an AOFAS score of 83.8 (95% CI 83.6–84.1) at a mean follow-up of13 years, but also found progression of radiographic degeneration in 28% of the cases.[52] At a mean of 6.3 years follow-up after bone marrow stimulation, Lambers observed that 54 out of 60 patients (90%) still participate in sports activities, of whom 53% at pre-injury level. However, they also observed that all the Foot and Ankle Outcome Scores (FAOS) significantly decreased between 1 year and final follow-up.[53]

Moses and colleagues conducted a retrospective study comparing 74 patients with OLT and CLAI with a matched group of 148 patients with OLT but without CLAI. Both groups underwent microfracture for the OLT, and lateral instability was addressed with anatomic repair. The 2 groups were matched in demographics and had similar VAS and AOFAS scores. At final follow-up (more than 50 months for both groups), they found comparable clinical outcomes in VAS, AOFAS, and all but 1 FAOS subtype score. The patients with CLAI had worse outcomes in the FAOS for the sport and recreation subscale, and the proportion of clinical failure was larger in this group when using an AOFAS score of less than 80 as the definition of failure (28.3% vs 16.2% in the non-CLAI group, $P = .03$)[54]

Another commonly performed procedure for OLT is the AMIC procedure. A recent meta-analysis evaluated the long-term outcomes of AMIC and found significant improvements in functional outcomes and pain scores. The meta-analysis included 12 studies with a total of 323 patients, and reported an improvement of 4.6 points in VAS, and 32.47 and 30.93 points in AOFAS and Foot Function Index, respectively. However, it should be noted that only half of the included studies specifically mentioned instability or malalignment in their cohorts. It remains unclear whether the patients included in these studies had no instability or malalignment, or if the authors did not assess these factors in their cohorts.[55] Several studies have specifically investigated the presence of instability in their cohorts; Richter and colleagues did specifically look for instability and found that the majority of patients in their cohort had concomitant instability. This resulted in 90% (130/144) of their patients undergoing a lateral stabilization procedure.[51] Similarly, Valderrabano found that 17 out of 26 patients with OLT had concomitant instability, requiring a ligamentous stabilization procedure. In another study by Wiewiorski, 41 out of 60 (68.3%) patients with OLT had ligamentous instability and underwent ligament repair.[5,56] These studies suggest that instability is a common finding in patients with OLT. More recently, Ackerman and colleagues conducted a retrospective study comparing 13 patients who underwent AMIC with concomitant lateral ligament stabilization (LLS) to a matched population of 83 patients who underwent isolated AMIC. They concluded that concurrent AMIC and LLS in patients with OLT and ankle instability results in a clinical outcome comparable to isolated AMIC if adequate postoperative ankle stability is achieved. However, residual ankle instability was associated with worse postoperative outcomes, highlighting the importance of achieving ankle stability in patients with OLT and concurrent ankle instability.[50] The importance of ankle stability was also demonstrated in a study by Kim, who investigated 27 patients with CAI and radiographic medial compartment osteoarthritis. After performing a lateral stabilization procedure, they found significant improvement in VAS score from 6.0 (SD 1.6) preoperatively to 1.8 (SD 1.6) postoperatively, AOFAS score from 61.9 (SD 14.2) to 89.7 (SD 6.2) and Karlsson–Peterson score from 54.7 (SD 13.9) to 88.3 (SD 9.0). The study demonstrated that even in patients with radiographic medial ankle osteoarthritis, ligament stabilization for individuals with CAI leads to improvement in functional outcomes with high patient satisfaction. However, whether the ligament stabilization procedure can slow or stop the progression of further osteoarthritis was not investigated[57]

POSTOPERATIVE CARE

When performing a surgical treatment for OLT along with a ligamentous stabilization procedure, it is important to consider a postoperative protocol that is applicable for both procedures. Different authors have used different postoperative protocols for treating lateral instability and OLT, and the ideal postoperative protocol remains a topic of debate.[46,48,51,58] In general, we apply a light non–weight baring cast for 2 weeks to allow for adequate wound healing. This is followed by 4 weeks in a removable walker boot, which permits active and passive range of motion in dorsiflexion and plantar flexion of the ankle to promote fibrocartilage and isometric ligamentous healing. Inversion should be prevented in the first 6 weeks to protect the lateral ligament stabilization. At 6 weeks post-surgery, we allow for the progressive removal of the walker boot and a return to full weight baring. While we are conservative in our postoperative weight baring protocol, it is worth noting that several studies have shown similar healing outcomes with both early and delayed weight bearing after bone marrow stimulation procedures.[59]

SUMMARY

Patients with an OLT typically present with deep ankle pain 6 to 12 months after an initial trauma. It is well known that both acute and chronic ankle instability cause pathologic stress on cartilage. While there are no comparative studies investigating the effect of stabilization procedures on cartilage repair, we believe that addressing instability is the key in the evaluation and treatment of an OLT. A personalized treatment plan should be developed, taking into account patient and OLT characteristics, associated injuries, and patient expectations. The "HALO" approach can be a helpful tool in the work up of OLT. It includes ankle stability and alignment as factors to consider in the treatment of OLT. We believe that failure to address these factors will lead to suboptimal outcomes of OLT treatment. After a surgical failure, it is important to start over and reassess all possible causes of the failure.

CLINICS CARE POINTS

- The majority of patients with an OLT present with a history of trauma. Typically, patients present with deep ankle pain 6 to 12 months after the initial trauma. Assessment for the presence of concurrent instability should be part of a routine examination in patients with OLT.

- When treating CLAI and OLT, no difference was found in patient outcomes between open and arthroscopic lateral stabilization procedures. Therefore, the choice of stabilization technique is dependent on the surgeons' preference.

- When determining the postoperative protocol after OLT and stabilization procedures, it is important to consider a protocol that is applicable to both procedures.

- When surgically treating instability and OLT, single-stage surgery shows similar results compared to a staged procedure. Therefore, a single-stage surgery is recommended.

- To our knowledge, there are no comparative studies investigating the effect of stabilization procedures on cartilage repair in patients with ankle instability. However, we believe that addressing instability is one of the key factors in a successful treatment of OLT.

DISCLOSURE

Competing interest: The authors declare no conflict of interest.

FUNDING

No funding was received for this article

REFERENCES

1. Donovan L, Hetzel S, Laufenberg CR, et al. Prevalence and Impact of Chronic Ankle Instability in Adolescent Athletes. Orthop J Sport Med 2020;8(2). 2325967119900962.
2. Krause F, Anwander H. Osteochondral lesion of the talus: still a problem? EFORT Open Rev 2022;7(6):337–43.
3. Kerkhoffs GMMJ, Kennedy JG, Calder JDF, et al. There is no simple lateral ankle sprain. Knee Surgery. Sport Traumatol Arthrosc 2016;24(4):941–3.
4. Hintermann B, Boss A, Schäfer D. Arthroscopic findings in patients with chronic ankle instability. Am J Sports Med 2002;30(3):402–9.
5. Wiewiorski M, Werner L, Paul J, et al. Sports Activity after Reconstruction of Osteochondral Lesions of the Talus with Autologous Spongiosa Grafts and Autologous Matrix-Induced Chondrogenesis. Am J Sports Med 2016;44(10):2651–8.

6. Valderrabano V, Hintermann B, Horisberger M, et al. Ligamentous posttraumatic ankle osteoarthritis. Am J Sports Med 2006;34(4):612–20.
7. Woods K, Harris I. Osteochondritis dissecans of the talus in identical twins. J Bone Joint Surg Br 1995;77(2):331.
8. Schachter AK, Chen AL, Reddy PD, et al. Osteochondral lesions of the talus. J Am Acad Orthop Surg 2005;13(3):152–8.
9. Choi WJ, Jo J, Lee JW. Osteochondral lesion of the talus: prognostic factors affecting the clinical outcome after arthroscopic marrow stimulation technique. Foot Ankle Clin 2013;18(1):67–78.
10. Mankin HJ. The response of articular cartilage to mechanical injury. J Bone Joint Surg Am 1982;64(3):460–6.
11. Zengerink M, Struijs PAA. Treatment of osteochondral lesions of the talus : a systematic review. Knee Surg Sports Arthrosc 2010;238–46.
12. Kerkhoffs GMMJ, Reilingh ML, Gerards RM, et al. Lift, drill, fill and fix (LDFF): a new arthroscopic treatment for talar osteochondral defects. Knee Surg Sports Traumatol Arthrosc 2016;24(4):1265–71.
13. Zwingmann J, Südkamp NP, Schmal H, et al. Surgical treatment of osteochondritis dissecans of the talus: A systematic review. Arch Orthop Trauma Surg 2012;132(9):1241–50.
14. Barnes CJ, Ferkel RD. Arthroscopic debridement and drilling of osteochondral lesions of the talus. Foot Ankle Clin 2003;8(2):243–57.
15. Giannini S, Buda R, Grigolo B, et al. Autologous chondrocyte transplantation in osteochondral lesions of the ankle joint. Foot Ankle Int 2001;22(6):513–7.
16. Ronga M, Grassi FA, Montoli C, Bulgheroni P, Genovese E, Cherubino P. Treatment of deep cartilage defects of the ankle with matrix-induced autologous chondrocyte implantation (MACI). Foot Ankle Surg (Internet). 2005;11(1):29–33. Available from: https://www.sciencedirect.com/science/article/pii/S1268773104000979.
17. Hangody L. The mosaicplasty technique for osteochondral lesions of the talus. Foot Ankle Clin 2003;8(2):259–73.
18. Imhoff AB, Paul J, Ottinger B, et al. Osteochondral transplantation of the talus: long-term clinical and magnetic resonance imaging evaluation. Am J Sports Med 2011;39(7):1487–93.
19. Close JR. Some applications of the functional anatomy of the ankle joint. J Bone Jt Surg [Am] 1956;761–81, 38-A.
20. Adelaar RS, Madrian JR. Avascular necrosis of the talus. Orthop Clin North Am 2004;35(3):383–95, xi.
21. Golanó P, Vega J, Leeuw PA de. Anatomy of the ankle ligaments: a pictorial essay. Knee Surg Sport Traumatol Arthrosc 2010;18:557–69.
22. Milner CE, Soames RW. Anatomical variations of the anterior talofibular ligament of the human ankle joint. J Anat 1997;191:457–8.
23. Ozeki S, Kitaoka H, Uchiyama E, et al. Ankle ligament tensile forces at the end points of passive circumferential rotating motion of the ankle and subtalar joint complex. Foot Ankle Int 2006;27(11):965–9.
24. Hunt KJ, Pereira H, Kelley J, et al. The Role of Calcaneofibular Ligament Injury in Ankle Instability: Implications for Surgical Management. Am J Sports Med 2019;47(2):431–7.
25. Brockett CL, Chapman GJ. Biomechanics of the ankle. Orthop Trauma (Internet). 2016;30(3):232–238. Available at: https://doi.org/10.1016/j.mporth.2016.04.015.
26. Lötscher P, Lang TH, Zwicky L, et al. Osteoligamentous injuries of the medial ankle joint. Eur J trauma Emerg Surg Off Publ Eur Trauma Soc 2015;41(6):615–21.

27. Ogilvie-Harris DJ, Reed SC, Hedman TP. Disruption of the ankle syndesmosis: biomechanical study of the ligamentous restraints. Arthrosc J Arthrosc Relat Surg Off Publ Arthrosc Assoc North Am Int Arthrosc Assoc 1994;10(5):558–60.

28. Corte-Real N, Caetano J. Ankle and syndesmosis instability: consensus and controversies. EFORT Open Rev 2021;6(6):420–31.

29. McKinley TO, Tochigi Y, Rudert MJ, et al. The effect of incongruity and instability on contact stress directional gradients in human cadaveric ankles. Osteoarthr Cartil 2008;16(11):1363–9.

30. Masson AO, Krawetz RJ. Understanding cartilage protection in OA and injury: a spectrum of possibilities. BMC Musculoskelet Disord 2020;21(1):432.

31. Welsch GH, Hennig FF, Krinner S, et al. T2 and T2* Mapping. Curr Radiol Rep 2014;2(8):1–9.

32. Trattnig S, Mamisch TC, Welsch GH, et al. Quantitative T2 mapping of matrix-associated autologous chondrocyte transplantation at 3 Tesla: an in vivo cross-sectional study. Invest Radiol 2007;42(6):442–8.

33. Tao H, Hu Y, Qiao Y, et al. T2-Mapping evaluation of early cartilage alteration of talus for chronic lateral ankle instability with isolated anterior talofibular ligament tear or combined with calcaneofibular ligament tear. J Magn Reson Imaging 2018;47(1):69–77.

34. Lee S, Yoon YC, Kim JH. T2 mapping of the articular cartilage in the ankle: Correlation to the status of anterior talofibular ligament. Clin Radiol [Internet] 2013; 68(7). e355–61.

35. Tao H, Zhang Y, Hu Y, et al. Cartilage Matrix Changes in Hindfoot Joints in Chronic Ankle Instability Patients After Anatomic Repair Using T2-Mapping: Initial Experience With 3-Year Follow-Up. J Magn Reson Imaging 2022;55(1):234–43.

36. Elias I, Zoga AC, Morrison WB, et al. Osteochondral lesions of the talus: localization and morphologic data from 424 patients using a novel anatomical grid scheme. Foot Ankle Int 2007;28(2):154–61.

37. Li X, Zhu Y, Xu Y, et al. Osteochondral autograft transplantation with biplanar distal tibial osteotomy for patients with concomitant large osteochondral lesion of the talus and varus ankle malalignment. BMC Musculoskelet Disord [Internet] 2017;18(1):23.

38. Knupp M, Pagenstert GI, Barg A, et al. SPECT-CT compared with conventional imaging modalities for the assessment of the varus and valgus malaligned hindfoot. J Orthop Res Off Publ Orthop Res Soc 2009;27(11):1461–6.

39. Loomer R, Fisher C, Lloyd-Smith R, et al. Osteochondral lesions of the talus. Am J Sports Med 1993;21(1):13–9.

40. Lan T, McCarthy HS, Hulme CH, et al. The management of talar osteochondral lesions - Current concepts. J Arthrosc Jt Surg [Internet] 2021;8(3):231–7.

41. Schmid MR, Pfirrmann CWA, Hodler J, et al. Cartilage lesions in the ankle joint: comparison of MR arthrography and CT arthrography. Skeletal Radiol 2003; 32(5):259–65.

42. Raheman FJ, Rojoa DM, Hallet C, Yaghmour KM, Jeyaparam S, Ahluwalia RS, et al. Can Weightbearing Cone-beam CT Reliably Differentiate Between Stable and Unstable Syndesmotic Ankle Injuries? A Systematic Review and Meta-analysis. Clin Orthop Relat Res (Internet). 2022;480(8). Available at: https://journals.lww.com/clinorthop/Fulltext/2022/08000/Can_Weightbearing_Cone_beam_CT_Reliably.21.aspx.

43. Pavani C, Belvedere C, Ortolani M, et al. 3D measurement techniques for the hindfoot alignment angle from weight-bearing CT in a clinical population. Sci Rep 2022;12(1):16900.

44. Allen T, Kelly M. Moder n Open and Minimally Invasive Stabilization of C h r o n i c L a t e r a l A n k l e I n s t a b i l i t y. Foot Ankle Clin NA 2023;26(1):87–101 [Internet].

45. Coughlin MJ, Schenck RCJ, Grebing BR, et al. Comprehensive reconstruction of the lateral ankle for chronic instability using a free gracilis graft. Foot Ankle Int 2004;25(4):231–41.

46. Jiang D, fang AY, Jiao C, et al. Concurrent arthroscopic osteochondral lesion treatment and lateral ankle ligament repair has no substantial effect on the outcome of chronic lateral ankle instability. Knee Surgery, Sport Traumatol Arthrosc [Internet] 2018;26(10):3129–34.

47. Feng SM, Chen J, Ma C, et al. Limited medial osteochondral lesions of the talus associated with chronic ankle instability do not impact the results of endoscopic modified Broström ligament repair. J Orthop Surg Res [Internet] 2022;17(1):1–8.

48. Xu C, Li M, Wang C, et al. A comparison between arthroscopic and open surgery for treatment outcomes of chronic lateral ankle instability accompanied by osteochondral lesions of the talus. J Orthop Surg Res 2020;15(1):1–9.

49. Wei Y, Song J, Yun X, et al. Outcomes of Single-Stage Versus Staged Treatment of Osteochondral Lesions in Patients With Chronic Lateral Ankle Instability: A Prospective Randomized Study. Orthop J Sport Med 2022;10(2):1–10.

50. Ackermann J, Casari FA, Germann C, et al. Autologous Matrix-Induced Chondrogenesis With Lateral Ligament Stabilization for Osteochondral Lesions of the Talus in Patients With Ankle Instability. Orthop J Sport Med 2021;9(5):1–7.

51. Richter M, Zech S, Andreas Meissner S. Matrix-associated stem cell transplantation (MAST) in chondral defects of the ankle is safe and effective – 2-year-followup in 130 patients. Foot Ankle Surg [Internet] 2017;23(4):236–42.

52. Rikken QGH, Dahmen J, Stufkens SAS, et al. Satisfactory long-term clinical outcomes after bone marrow stimulation of osteochondral lesions of the talus. Knee Surgery. Sport Traumatol Arthrosc [Internet] 2021;29(11):3525–33.

53. Lambers KTA, Dahmen J, Altink JN, et al. Bone marrow stimulation for talar osteochondral lesions at long-term follow-up shows a high sports participation though a decrease in clinical outcomes over time. Knee Surgery, Sport Traumatol Arthrosc [Internet] 2021;29(5):1562–9.

54. Lee M, Kwon JW, Choi WJ, et al. Comparison of Outcomes for Osteochondral Lesions of the Talus with and Without Chronic Lateral Ankle Instability. Foot Ankle Int 2015;36(9):1050–7.

55. Walther M, Valderrabano V, Wiewiorski M, et al. Is there clinical evidence to support autologous matrix-induced chondrogenesis (AMIC) for chondral defects in the talus? A systematic review and meta-analysis. Foot Ankle Surg [Internet] 2021;27(3):236–45.

56. Valderrabano V, Miska M, Leumann A, et al. Reconstruction of osteochondral lesions of the talus with autologous spongiosa grafts and autologous matrix-induced chondrogenesis. Am J Sports Med 2013;41(3):519–27.

57. Kim SW, Jung HG, Lee JS. Ligament stabilization improved clinical and radiographic outcomes for individuals with chronic ankle instability and medial ankle osteoarthritis. Knee Surgery, Sport Traumatol Arthrosc [Internet] 2020;28(10): 3294–300.

58. Yasui Y, Takao M, Miyamoto W, et al. Simultaneous surgery for chronic lateral ankle instability accompanied by only subchondral bone lesion of talus. Arch Orthop Trauma Surg 2014;134(6):821–7.

59. Song M, Li S, Yang S, et al. Is Early or Delayed Weightbearing the Better Choice After Microfracture for Osteochondral Lesions of the Talus? A Meta-analysis and Systematic Review. J Foot Ankle Surg [Internet] 2021;60(6):1232–40.

Deformity Correction
Do Osteochondral Lesion of the Talus and Tibia Change After Realignment Surgery?

Jaeyoung Kim, MD[a], Woo-Chun Lee, MD, PhD[b],*

KEYWORDS

- Osteochondral lesion • Talus • Realignment surgery • Supramalleolar • Osteotomy
- Malalignment • Cyst • OLT

KEY POINTS

- Increased contact stress on a specific area within the ankle joint is one of the proposed etiologies of osteochondral lesions of the talus (OLTs).
- Malalignment of the foot, ankle, and lower limb can alter ankle joint kinematics, potentially leading to the development of the OLT.
- Realignment surgery has been shown to have a positive impact on cartilage lesions in the knee joint in a decent amount of research.
- Although data is still limited, there is promising evidence that isolated realignment surgery in the ankle joint can lead to improved patient symptoms and radiographic profile of the OLT.

INTRODUCTION

The pathogenesis of osteochondral lesions of the talus (OLTs) and tibia is not yet fully understood. Although OLTs can develop following a traumatic event,[1] some cases occur spontaneously, and bilateral presentations with no prior trauma are not uncommon.[2,3] Increased contact stress on a specific area within the ankle joint is one of the proposed etiologies for the development or progression of OLTs.[4] Therefore, it is logical to evaluate the possible root causes of such eccentric load within the ankle joint and address them to optimize surgical outcomes. However, current surgical strategies for patients with OLT primarily focus on treating the affected lesion,[5,6] either repairing or replacing it, with limited attention paid to the biomechanical environment of the ankle joint.

[a] Foot and Ankle Service, Hospital for Special Surgery, 532 East 72nd Street, New York, NY, USA;
[b] Seoul Foot and Ankle Center, Dubalo Orthopaedic Clinic, 45, Apgujeong-ro 30 gil, Gangnam-gu, Seoul 06022, Republic of Korea
* Corresponding author.
E-mail address: leewoochun@gmail.com

Foot Ankle Clin N Am 29 (2024) 333–342
https://doi.org/10.1016/j.fcl.2023.07.006

Malalignment can significantly affect ankle joint biomechanics, leading to increased eccentric pressure within the joint.[7,8] Unaddressed malalignment of the foot and ankle has been proposed as a potential cause of OLT surgery failure,[9] and there is growing recognition of the association between malalignment and OLTs.[9–11] Although the literature describes "normal" or "physiologic" alignment as a prerequisite for successful cartilage surgery and advocates for the correction of malalignment as a first step,[12,13] there is a paucity of data on the outcomes of realignment surgery in patients with OLT.

This article aims to elucidate the rationale behind realignment surgery in patients with OLT, as well as outcomes reported in the literature, in order to shed light on an important but thus far unexplored area of the efficacy of realignment surgery in patients with OLT.

Possible Association Between the Malalignment and Development of Osteochondral Lesions of the Talus

Despite the lack of conclusive evidence on the direct causal relationship between malalignment and the development of osteochondral lesions of the talus (OLTs), there is widespread recognition that eccentric forces within specific areas of the ankle joint can produce excessive contact stress, potentially leading to cartilage damage and subchondral bone changes.[10,13] Malalignment of the lower limb, including the hindfoot, has been identified as a known cause of altered load distribution patterns within the ankle joint,[7,8,14–16] and therefore, may increase an individual's susceptibility to OLTs.

Several theories have been proposed to explain the development of OLTs, with increased focal pressure on the specific area of the talus being considered as an important initiator or contributor. One popular theory suggests that increased focal stress can lead to cartilage degeneration, crack formation, and exacerbate lesions by creating a check-valve effect that increases hydrostatic pressure within the subchondral bone.[17] Another theory proposes that OLTs may be a physiologic adaptive response of cartilage and subchondral bone to focal stress in accordance with Wolff's law.[18] This theory may account for instances where the cartilage cover remains intact despite the presence of a cyst at the subchondral lesion. Finally, overloading may induce poor vascularization due to osseous hypertension, resulting in chondrocyte metabolism suppression and decreased collagen biosynthesis.[19,20] These factors may impede the regeneration of injured cartilage, and suggest that malalignment may negatively impact healing even in post-traumatic OLTs.

Location of Deformity

The effect of coronal plane distal tibial deformities, such as varus or valgus orientation, on ankle joint pressure has been the subject of various studies using cadaveric specimens. In one study, Knupp and colleagues investigated intra-articular pressure after creating supramalleolar varus and valgus deformities.[7] Their findings demonstrated that the tibia osteotomy with concomitant fibular osteotomy resulted in a change in the center of force and peak pressure in the anteromedial direction after varus angulation, and in the posterolateral direction after valgus angulation.[7] The simultaneous anteroposterior direction changes in joint pressure suggests that the coronal plane deformity may act on the ankle joint in a multiplanar action, with the potential for a similar effect from supramalleolar osteotomy (SMO). Another study by Schmid and colleagues found that a lateral closing wedge SMO in a fixed cavovarus model reduced anteromedial ankle joint contact stresses.[8] While not specific to patients with OLT, clinical observational studies have indicated that SMO results in a significant clinical and radiographic improvement in patients with ankle arthritis.[8] All above findings suggest that the SMO shifts the load to the contralateral side, potentially unloading the talus and tibia in the affected area.

The impact of hindfoot alignment on ankle joint load distribution patterns and kinematics has also been demonstrated in several biomechanical studies. Michelson and colleagues found that medial displacement calcaneal osteotomy can increase ankle varus and internal rotation at the ankle joint in dorsiflexed position.[16] While the absolute values of change in kinematics were relatively small, even minor changes in ankle kinematics may significantly affect pressure distribution within the ankle joint. Similarly, Steffensmeier and colleagues demonstrated that the center of force in the ankle moved slightly medial or lateral following a 1 cm displacement osteotomy in the corresponding direction.[21] They also found that local regions in the ankle joint were unloaded after the calcaneus was shifted in the opposite direction. Davitt and colleagues showed similar results that the center of force moves medially with a medial displacement osteotomy and laterally with a lateral displacement osteotomy.[15]

However, caution is needed when interpreting these findings and incorporating them into OLT patient treatment, as the aforementioned cadaveric studies were conducted on normal arched specimens, and the effect of calcaneal osteotomy may differ in patients with malalignment whose kinematics of talus is already different than those of normal patients. For instance, in patients with flatfoot deformity, the talus may internally rotate,[22,23] thereby increasing medial tibiotalar joint pressure. Our clinical experience suggests that the correction of flatfoot deformity may alleviate medial side symptoms, as well as improve radiographic profile of medial side osteochondral lesions (**Fig. 1**). Therefore, it can be argued that improving the overall biomechanical

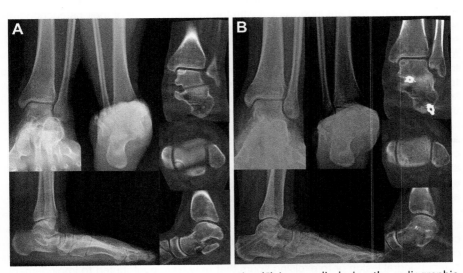

Fig. 1. Preoperative (*A*) and 5-year postoperative (*B*) images displaying the radiographic changes in a patient with a large posteromedial osteochondral lesion of the talus (OLT), who also presented with a flatfoot deformity. The OLT exhibits an improved radiographic profile following the correction of the flatfoot deformity through subtalar arthrodesis and dynamic medial column stabilization (achieved via flexor hallucis longus tendon transfer to the first metatarsal). Notably, this improvement is observed without any direct intervention specifically targeting the OLT.

environment may not only relieve patient symptoms, but also have a positive impact on osteochondral lesions.

Another theory explaining potential role of foot alignment exists. Ikuta and colleagues investigated foot alignment in pediatric patients with nontraumatic medial OLTs.[24] They found that those with medial OLT have low medial longitudinal arch compared to those of control patients.[24] Also, they found that the attachment of deep deltoid ligament was more proximally located in the medial OLT group compared to controls.[24] They hypothesized that increased medial traction force of the deep deltoid fiber both from the location of it as well as valgus hindfoot may be associated with the development of the talar dome lesion.

Furthermore, whole lower limb alignment plays a crucial role in ankle joint load distribution.[25,26] Even with a neutral orientation of the distal tibial plafond to the tibial axis, varus or valgus lower limb mechanical axis can induce altered kinematics, as observed in previous studies.[26]

Why We Consider Realignment Procedures in Patients with Osteochondral Lesions of the Talus?

Which symptom characterizes OLT, and to what extent do the lesions explain the diverse symptoms reported by patients in the clinic? OLT commonly presents with vague, poorly defined symptoms at the ankle joint, and there may be a discrepancy between the lesion location and the site of pain and symptoms in affected patients. The published literature on OLT and surgical outcomes tends to overlook the clinical presentation of the patients and instead emphasizes radiographic features of the lesion, such as location, size, depth, and cartilage appearance on magnetic resonance imaging (MRI).

In our clinical experience, a substantial proportion of patients with OLT describe primary symptoms that are inconsistent with the location or size of their osteochondral lesions. Rather, they present with an array of mechanical impingement symptoms, either at the ankle joint or sinus tarsi. For instance, patients with a posteromedial lesion may report lateral-sided pain as their primary symptom. While some have proposed that this phenomenon results from an inflammatory response in the ankle joint leading to synovitis and diffuse ankle symptoms, we have observed that many patients with lateral side pain experience pain at the sinus tarsi, an extra-articular location outside the ankle joint. This sinus tarsi impingement suggests that there may be a subtle subluxation at the subtalar joint,[27] leading to aberrant talar motion within the ankle mortise and this may not improve with a cartilage procedure alone. Therefore, we posit that the correction of alignment should take precedence after carefully examining patients about their symptoms. By addressing the underlying abnormal kinematics of the ankle, the symptoms of patients with OLT may be better relieved than by solely addressing the lesion itself if concurrent malalignment exists.

Spur formation in the ankle joint in patients with OLT may provide further evidence of the involvement of altered kinematics in their development or progression. As concomitant spur excision is commonly performed during OLT surgery, it remains unclear whether symptomatic improvement is primarily attributable to addressing the osteochondral lesion or to excising spurs that may have contributed to impingement symptoms. Spur formation in the ankle joint could be the result of abnormal ankle kinematics leading to impingement or tight triceps surae, resulting in limited dorsiflexion of the ankle joint when viewed from a different perspective.[28]

Moreover, the conventional understanding of normal alignment warrants re-evaluation. While weightbearing ankle radiographs have traditionally been used to assess alignment, our clinical experience suggests that weightbearing computed tomography (WBCT) reveals subtle joint space narrowing or talus tilting in some patients with OLT that may impact ankle biomechanics, even in the absence of radiographic abnormalities in plain radiographs.

Based on these observations, we postulate that altered joint kinematics may contribute to the pathogenesis and progression of OLT and the associated symptoms in patients. Therefore, we maintain that solely addressing the lesion may not be sufficient to fully alleviate the symptoms of patients with OLT. A comprehensive assessment of the patient's symptoms and examination of the underlying kinematics should be taken into account when determining the most appropriate treatment plan.

What to Look at and Assess in Radiographs?

Weightbearing radiographs are a crucial tool for assessing concurrent foot and ankle deformities. In weightbearing ankle anteroposterior views, coronal plane distal tibia orientation is typically assessed using the medial distal tibia angle (MDTA), and talar tilt (TT) angle is evaluated to determine if there is focal narrowing of the tibiotalar joint. Additionally, the mediolateral position of the talus relative to the tibial axis is considered an important indicator of medial or lateral shear force within the ankle mortise, as some ankles do not tilt but instead translate in the coronal plane. This position is assessed using talar center migration (TCM), as previously described.[26,29–32]

In weightbearing foot radiographs, common flatfoot parameters such as the talonavicular coverage angle (TNC), lateral talo-1st metatarsal (Meary's) angle, and calcaneal pitch (CP) are evaluated.[33]

In hindfoot alignment views, both the hindfoot moment arm and hindfoot alignment angle are measured to assess hindfoot alignment. This is due to the fact that the hindfoot can often demonstrate translation without a corresponding degree of angulation, or vice versa.

In our clinical practice, WBCT plays an important role, providing a more comprehensive explanation for undergoing realignment procedures than plain radiographs alone. For patients with lateral-sided pain, sinus tarsi impingement, or calcaneofibular impingement can be assessed, and this may warrant realignment procedures as these findings may not improve with direct procedures for OLTs. Additionally, our experience suggests a discrepancy between plain radiographs and WBCT in terms of distal tibial plafond orientation relative to the tibial axis or talar tilt. Furthermore, many patients who have normal-looking ankles on plain radiographs exhibit slight narrowing of the joint space in WBCT, indicating that the correction of an altered biomechanical environment may improve patient symptoms.

Can Improvement of Biomechanical Environment Improve Cartilage Lesion?

Realignment surgery and its effects on cartilage regeneration in the ankle joint have not been extensively studied. However, several studies have explored this phenomenon in patients with knee compartment arthritis, which suggest that realignment surgery alone may improve the cartilage profile.

Jung and colleagues reviewed patients who had undergone high tibial osteotomy (HTO) for medial compartment osteoarthritis and found cartilage regeneration even without cartilage regeneration procedures during second-look arthroscopy.[34] They also discovered that those with mechanical tibiofemoral angle within the "ideal" range (0–6°) after surgery had more frequent cartilage regeneration than those with overcorrection or undercorrection, highlighting the importance of proper alignment in cartilage regeneration.[34] Similarly, Koshino and colleagues reported partial or total cartilage regeneration in 133 out of 146 knees that underwent high tibial osteotomy without chondrocyte implantation or drilling, suggesting a possible association between limb alignment and articular cartilage status.[35] Wang and colleagues found that malalignment is associated with more frequent cyst formation, as demonstrated by spontaneous regression of subchondral bone cysts in patients with knee osteoarthritis who underwent HTO and were followed up using MRI after 5 years.[18]

In the case of focal cartilage defects in the knee joint, Farber and colleagues found that performing realignment surgery alongside cartilage procedures leads to better postoperative patient-reported outcome scores, lower pain levels, and higher patient satisfaction compared to cartilage procedures alone.[36]

Regarding the ankle joint, a study by Jung and colleagues found improved cartilage profile in 12 out of 14 ankles 1 year after surgery in patients who had SMOs for varus ankle arthritis.[37] Although this study was not specific to patients with OLT, it suggests that realignment surgery may have a positive effect on cartilage regeneration in the ankle joint, particularly in cases where focal pressure is relieved.

Outcomes of Osteochondral Lesions of the Talus Procedure Together with Realignment Surgery

Li and colleagues reported successful outcomes in 11 cases where biplanar SMO was performed concurrently with OATs for patients with a large OLT and varus distal tibial deformity.[11] Similarly, Wiewiorski and colleagues described a case in which SMO with flatfoot reconstruction was performed in a patient who had failed OATs and had concurrent valgus distal tibial plafond and flatfoot deformity.[38] Slullitel and colleagues presented successful treatment of a lateral OLT in a pediatric patient with allograft transplantation, together with coalition resection and hindfoot realignment surgery.[39] They surmised that their successful 2-year follow-up outcome may be, in part, due to the realigned hindfoot, which avoids overloading over the implanted allograft.[39] Although these studies suggest the potential benefits of realignment surgery in patients with OLT, the isolated effect of realignment surgery on the healing of osteochondral lesions has not been fully elucidated.

Outcomes of Isolated Realignment Surgery in Patients with Osteochondral Lesions of the Talus

Currently, only two studies have investigated the effects of isolated realignment surgery in patients with OLT. Kim and colleagues reported on eight patients who had previously undergone OAT but having persistent pain and subsequently developed cystic lesions around the plug.[9] There were notable malalignment at the distal tibia or hindfoot. Despite not directly treating the osteochondral lesion, the patients experienced both clinical and radiographic improvements in their condition after undergoing realignment procedures.[9]

In another recent study, Kim and colleagues examined the effects of isolated realignment surgery in patients with large cystic osteochondral lesions and malalignment.[40] The study included 27 patients with large cystic osteochondral lesions of the talar shoulder, for which fresh allograft transplantation had been recommended due to the lesion's uncontained nature. They found that the patients in the cohort demonstrated symptoms that does not match the location of the osteochondral lesion, and many of them described sinus tarsi pain as their primary location of pain. With the hypothesis that patients in the cohort experienced symptoms more indicative of malalignment, the authors performed realignment procedures rather than addressing osteochondral lesion. Following realignment procedures, the patients showed improvements in their functional outcome scores, and surprisingly, there was radiographic evidence of improvement in the cystic osteochondral lesions. The report

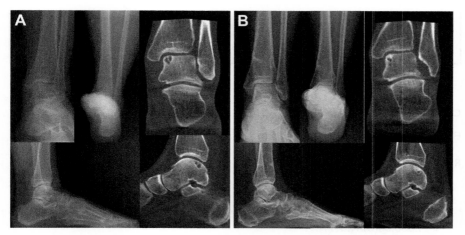

Fig. 2. Preoperative (A) and 7-year postoperative (B) images showing the radiographic changes of a large posteromedial osteochondral lesion of the talus (OLT) in a patient concurrently presenting with a varus distal tibial plafond. The OLT demonstrates an improved radiographic profile following the medial opening wedge supramalleolar osteotomy and medial displacement calcaneal osteotomy.

was based on a mean follow-up of 4.1 years, during which no patients required subsequent surgery aimed at the osteochondral lesion.

Although it is based on our unpublished data, we have noted a significant improvement in patient-reported outcomes and radiographic profiles of OLTs after isolated realignment surgery (**Fig. 2**). Additionally, it is a rare occurrence for those patients to require additional procedures to address OLTs. These findings prompt us to consider whether the lesion itself is the primary source of the pain that patients report, or if we have overlooked the importance of the biomechanical environment in patients with OLT.

SUMMARY

Although there is still limited evidence on the consistent effectiveness of realignment procedures for improving osteochondral lesions of the talus and tibia, the available literature suggests that realignment may be a reasonable approach for patients with OLT, particularly those with discernible malalignment or symptoms associated with malalignment. Despite the advancements made in tissue engineering and orthoregeneration, a biomechanically sound environment of the ankle joint, achieved through acceptable foot, ankle, and hindfoot alignment, remains a crucial prerequisite for the successful treatment of OLTs. Further studies are needed to confirm the efficacy of realignment procedures in this context.

CLINICS CARE POINTS

- Malalignment can significantly affect ankle joint biomechanics, leading to an increased eccentric pressure within the joint. This pressure can be a cause of the development of osteochondral lesions in the ankle joint.

- Simultaneous correction of malalignment has been proven to yield better patient outcomes compared to isolated cartilage surgery in patients with knee joint cartilage defects.

> • There is mounting evidence in the ankle joint that concurrent correction of malalignment in addition to cartilage repair or isolated malalignment correction would result in favorable outcomes for patients with osteochondral lesions of the talus.

CONFLICT OF INTEREST

Both authors have nothing to disclose pertaining to this topic.

REFERENCES

1. Kraeutler MJ, Chahla J, Dean CS, et al. Current concepts review update: osteochondral lesions of the talus. Foot Ankle Int 2017;38(3):331–42.
2. Hermanson E, Ferkel RD. Bilateral osteochondral lesions of the talus. Foot Ankle Int 2009;30(8):723–7.
3. Rikken QG, Wolsink LM, Dahmen J, et al. 15% of Talar Osteochondral Lesions Are Present Bilaterally While Only 1 in 3 Bilateral Lesions Are Bilaterally Symptomatic. JBJS 2022;104(18):1605–13.
4. Knupp M, Pagenstert GI, Barg A, et al. SPECT-CT compared with conventional imaging modalities for the assessment of the varus and valgus malaligned hindfoot. J Orthop Res 2009;27(11):1461–6.
5. Steele JR, Dekker TJ, Federer AE, et al. Osteochondral lesions of the talus: current concepts in diagnosis and treatment. Foot & Ankle Orthopaedics 2018;3(3). 2473011418779559.
6. Hurley ET, Murawski CD, Paul J, et al. Osteochondral autograft: proceedings of the international consensus meeting on cartilage repair of the ankle. Foot Ankle Int 2018;39(1_suppl):28S–34S.
7. Knupp M, Stufkens SA, van Bergen CJ, et al. Effect of supramalleolar varus and valgus deformities on the tibiotalar joint: a cadaveric study. Foot Ankle Int 2011; 32(6):609–15.
8. Schmid T, Zurbriggen S, Zderic I, et al. Ankle joint pressure changes in a pes cavovarus model: supramalleolar valgus osteotomy versus lateralizing calcaneal osteotomy. Foot Ankle Int 2013;34(9):1190–7.
9. Kim J, Rajan L, Gagne O, et al. Realignment Surgery for Failed Osteochondral Autologous Transplantation in Osteochondral Lesions of the Talus Associated With Malalignment. Foot Ankle Spec 2023. https://doi.org/10.1177/19386400231163030. 19386400231163030.
10. Easley ME, Vineyard JC. Varus ankle and osteochondral lesions of the talus. Foot Ankle Clin 2012;17(1):21–38.
11. Li X, Zhu Y, Xu Y, et al. Osteochondral autograft transplantation with biplanar distal tibial osteotomy for patients with concomitant large osteochondral lesion of the talus and varus ankle malalignment. BMC Muscoskel Disord 2017; 18(1):1–10.
12. Bazaz R, Ferkel RD. Treatment of osteochondral lesions of the talus with autologous chondrocyte implantation. Tech Foot Ankle Surg 2004;3(1):45–52.
13. Reilingh M, Van Bergen C, Van Dijk C. Diagnosis and treatment of osteochondral defects of the ankle. SA Orthopaedic Journal 2009;8(2):44–50.
14. Krause FG, Sutter D, Waehnert D, et al. Ankle joint pressure changes in a pes cavovarus model after lateralizing calcaneal osteotomies. Foot Ankle Int 2010; 31(9):741–6.

15. Davitt JS, Beals TC, Bachus KN. The effects of medial and lateral displacement calcaneal osteotomies on ankle and subtalar joint pressure distribution. Foot Ankle Int 2001;22(11):885–9.

16. Michelson JD, Mizel M, Jay P, et al. Effect of medial displacement calcaneal osteotomy on ankle kinematics in a cadaver model. Foot Ankle Int 1998;19(3): 132–6.

17. Van Dijk CN, Reilingh ML, Zengerink M, et al. Osteochondral defects in the ankle: why painful? Knee Surg Sports Traumatol Arthrosc 2010;18:570–80.

18. Wang W, Ding R, Zhang N, et al. Subchondral bone cysts regress after correction of malalignment in knee osteoarthritis: comply with Wolff's law. Int Orthop 2021; 45:445–51.

19. Buschmann MD, Hunziker EB, Kim Y-J, et al. Altered aggrecan synthesis correlates with cell and nucleus structure in statically compressed cartilage. J Cell Sci 1996;109(2):499–508.

20. Arnoldi CC, Lemperg RK, Linderholm H, et al. Intraosseous hypertension and pain in the knee. Journal of Bone and Joint Surgery British 1975;57(3):360–3.

21. Steffensmeier S, Berbaum K, Brown T. Effects of medial and lateral displacement calcaneal osteotomies on tibiotalar joint contact stresses. J Orthop Res 1996; 14(6):980–5.

22. Kim J, Rajan L, Henry J, et al. Axial plane rotation of the talus in progressive collapsing foot deformity: A weightbearing computed tomography analysis. Foot Ankle Int 2023;44(4):281–90.

23. Henry JK, Hoffman J, Kim J, et al. The Foot and Ankle Kinematics of a Simulated Progressive Collapsing Foot Deformity During Stance Phase: A Cadaveric Study. Foot Ankle Int 2022;43(12):1577–86.

24. Ikuta Y, Nakasa T, Sumii J, et al. Radiographic foot alignment and morphological features of deltoid ligament in pediatric patients with medial osteochondral lesions of the talus. J Pediatr Orthop B 2023;32(1):39–46.

25. Haraguchi N, Ota K, Tsunoda N, et al. Weight-bearing-line analysis in supramalleolar osteotomy for varus-type osteoarthritis of the ankle. JBJS 2015;97(4): 333–9.

26. Kim J, Henry JK, Kim J-B, et al. Dome supramalleolar osteotomies for the treatment of ankle pain with opposing coronal plane deformities between ankle and the lower limb. Foot Ankle Int 2022;43(4):474–85.

27. Kim J, Rajan L, Fuller R, et al. Radiographic cutoff values for predicting lateral bony impingement in progressive collapsing foot deformity. Foot Ankle Int 2022;43(9):1219–26.

28. Talusan PG, Toy J, Perez JL, et al. Anterior ankle impingement: diagnosis and treatment. J Am Acad Orthop Surg 2014;22(5):333–9.

29. Yi Y, Cho J-H, Kim J-B, et al. Change in talar translation in the coronal plane after mobile-bearing total ankle replacement and its association with lower-limb and hindfoot alignment. JBJS 2017;99(4):e13.

30. Kim J, Kim J-B, Lee W-C. Eccentric ankle arthritis in the sagittal plane: a novel description of anterior and posterior ankle arthritis. Foot Ankle Surg 2021;27(8): 934–41.

31. Kim J, Kim J-B, Lee W-C. Outcomes of joint preservation surgery in valgus ankle arthritis without deltoid ligament insufficiency. Foot Ankle Int 2021;42(11): 1419–30.

32. Kim J-B, Park CH, Ahn J-Y, et al. Characteristics of medial gutter arthritis on weightbearing CT and plain radiograph. Skeletal Radiol 2021;50:1575–83.

33. Younger AS, Sawatzky B, Dryden P. Radiographic assessment of adult flatfoot. Foot Ankle Int 2005;26(10):820–5.
34. Jung W-H, Takeuchi R, Chun C-W, et al. Second-look arthroscopic assessment of cartilage regeneration after medial opening-wedge high tibial osteotomy. Arthroscopy 2014;30(1):72–9.
35. Koshino T, Wada S, Ara Y, et al. Regeneration of degenerated articular cartilage after high tibial valgus osteotomy for medial compartmental osteoarthritis of the knee. Knee 2003;10(3):229–36.
36. Faber S, Angele P, Zellner J, et al. Comparison of Clinical Outcome following Cartilage Repair for Patients with Underlying Varus Deformity with or without Additional High Tibial Osteotomy: A Propensity Score–Matched Study Based on the German Cartilage Registry (KnorpelRegister DGOU). Cartilage 2021; 13(1_suppl):1206S–16S.
37. Jung H-G, Lee D-O, Lee S-H, et al. Second-look arthroscopic evaluation and clinical outcome after supramalleolar osteotomy for medial compartment ankle osteoarthritis. Foot Ankle Int 2017;38(12):1311–7.
38. Wiewiorski M, Miska M, Nicolas G, et al. Revision of failed osteochondral autologous transplantation procedure for chronic talus osteochondral lesion with iliac crest graft and autologous matrix-induced chondrogenesis: a case report. Foot Ankle Spec 2012;5(2):115–20.
39. Slullitel PA, Tripodi ML, Bosio ST, et al. Massive osteochondral lesion of the talus in a skeletally immature patient associated with a tarsal coalition and valgus hindfoot. J Foot Ankle Surg 2017;56(6):1257–62.
40. Kim J, Yi Y, Lee WC. Isolated realignment surgery improves clinical and radiographic outcomes in patients with large cystic osteochondral lesion of the talar shoulder with concurrent malalignment, Orthop J Sports Med, In press.

Fresh Osteochondral Allograft for Large Talar Osteochondral Lesions

Christopher Edward Gross, MD[a], Ariel Palanca, MD[b],*

KEYWORDS

- Osteochondral lesions • Talus OCD • Talar OCD • Hemitalar allograft • OLT

KEY POINTS

- Lesions which are large (>1 cm), located in the medial or lateral talar shoulder or incongruously shaped, typically require a structural graft.
- The key benefits of allograft transplantation include no donor site morbidity and the need for only one surgery. Furthermore, it affords the ability to handle large defects and to specifically match the curvature of the cartilage surface.
- A surgeon's approach is dictated by the location and size of the lesion.

INTRODUCTION

Osteochondral lesions of the talus (OLTs) are a common pathology of the ankle joint and are often associated with ankle injuries. Rates of OLTs have been reported in 50% to 73% of acute ankle injuries[1,2] and up to 88% of patients who sustain an ankle fracture.[3,4] OLTs can also be noninjury-related and can be caused by several different pathologies including genetic predisposition, degenerative joint disease, avascular necrosis, or patient-specific factors such as peripheral vascular disease.[5] The consensus is there is no need to operatively treat asymptomatic OLTs. Several retrospective studies have shown good results with conservative treatment for nondisplaced OLTs with a reported a 45% to 89% success rate using conservative treatment based on preoperative symptomatology.[6–8] However, in symptomatic patients, surgery is often indicated for symptom resolution.

A variety of techniques have been reported for the treatment of OLTs.[6,9–11] The successful treatment of OLTs can be challenging given the retrograde blood supply of the talus, the considerable forces transmitted through the ankle joint, and a low density of chondrocyte progenitor cells.[12]

[a] Department of Orthopaedics, Medical University of South Carolina, Charleston, SC 29403, USA; [b] Department of Orthopaedics, Palomar Health Medical Group, 15611 Pomerado Road, Poway, CA 92064, USA
* Corresponding author.
E-mail address: Ariel.palanca@gmail.com

Foot Ankle Clin N Am 29 (2024) 343–356
https://doi.org/10.1016/j.fcl.2023.07.009
1083-7515/24/© 2023 Elsevier Inc. All rights reserved.

foot.theclinics.com

Smaller lesions can be treated with arthroscopic debridement plus or minus bone marrow stimulation (microfracture), as a means of inducing fibrocartilage growth consisting primarily of type I and type III collagen rather than the typical type II collagen of hyaline cartilage.[13] Satisfactory results have been reported in more than 80% of the patients[4] in the short term; however, recent literature questions the long-term efficacy of this procedure.[14,15]

After debridement, some industry companies now offer forms of nonautologous grafts, including extracellular matrix and particulated juvenile cartilage. Other graft substitutes have a small osseous layer as well to substitute for mild bone loss and to allow bone-to-bone healing. These grafts can be secured by fibrin glue or a suture anchor. Autologous chondrocyte implantation (ACI) is a technique which provides an autologous cartilage graft to the defect but requires two surgeries—the first to harvest the chondrocytes and the second to implant after growth. The use of biologics as an adjunct is common, with reported improved results.[16,17] The most used biologic adjuncts include concentrated bone marrow aspirate, platelet-rich plasma, hyaluronic acid, and micronized adipose tissue.[18,19]

Lesions which are large (>1 cm), located in the medial or lateral talar shoulder, or incongruously shaped, typically require a structural graft. The current treatment techniques include osteochondral autograft transfer (OATS)/mosaicplasty from the knee and osteochondral allograft transplantation. If using OATS for large lesions, one can nestle two lesions side by side or adjunct with cancellous graft.[20]

The key benefits of allograft transplantation include no donor site morbidity and the need for only one surgery. Furthermore, it affords the ability to handle large defects and to specifically match the curvature of the cartilage surface. One study reviewed talar specimens after failed microfracture for an OLT which later underwent fresh osteochondral allograft transplantation. The microfractured tali showed significantly worse quality of bone as well as surface smoothness compared with the allograft, along with increased cytokines and matrix metalloproteinases (MMPs).[21] Another benefit of allograft transplantation over OATS is a more reliable and quicker return to sport and active duty.[22]

Cartilage viability is required for successful clinical outcomes after transplantation of osteochondral allografts, so storage and handling are very important. The allograft can be stored frozen or fresh. Fresh allografts have shown better results in terms of cellular viability, stiffness, and matrix content both at the time of implantation and longer term follow-up.[23] The length of storage can also affect chondrocyte viability, as declination of properties can be seen at 28 days.[24] Furthermore, damage can be seen both to the allograft and the recipient talus at the time of implantation if not handled properly. Given the variability between tissue banks for storage, testing, and procurement, there is potential for future research regarding the proper choice of storage medium, temperature, and use of adjust in the serum such as insulin growth factor-1.[25]

Currently, fresh osteochondral allografts are used in clinical practice, but the recommendation for storage length varies widely between authors, ranging from 24 to 48 hours to 2 weeks, or even longer.[24,26] Fresh osteochondral allografts in the knee have been shown to contain viable chondrocytes for up to 17 years after transplantation in one study; however, other studies refute that data showing no viable chondrocytes at 1 year after transplantation.[26–29]

INDICATIONS AND CONTRAINDICATIONS

Acute displaced OLTs in the setting of injury are usually treated by excision followed by chondroplasty and possible microfracture or a cartilage graft. The repair of large fragments has been reported, particularly in juveniles with an intact cartilage surface.[30] Conservative management of chronic lesions is often successful, so nonoperative management is the first line of treatment for nondisplaced chronic lesions. The failure of nonoperative management (continued pain, mechanical symptoms, or ability to return to sport) is an indication for surgery.

Typically, patients with minimally symptomatic nondisplaced OLTs[31,32] are initially treated with a trial of 3 to 6 months of nonsurgical management. There is not a strong recommendation of an appropriate nonoperative protocol for OLTs, but typical treatment includes anti-inflammatories and analgesics, activity modification, and protected weight-bearing with immobilization.

Initial surgical treatment for small, contained lesions should include some form of debridement, curettage, or microfracture, so there is a stable bleeding base. Failed initial debridement is an indication for resurfacing, as in OATS, ACI, or structural allograft. Generally, osteochondral allograft transplantation is not first-line treatment unless the lesion is large (>1.5 cm) or a shoulder lesion as allograft can be shaped to address different locations and different lesion sizes. Plug-shaped allografts or block-shaped allografts can be used based on the defect.

Contraindications for surgery include degenerative joint disease or an active infection. In the setting of malalignment or ligamentous laxity, these problems need to be addressed either before an allograft transplantation or concurrently.[23]

Planning

Preoperative planning includes obtaining x-rays, a CT scan, an MRI, and a SPECT-CT scan to define the location, size, cartilage surface, and joint condition. Plain x-rays include weight-bearing antero-posterior, lateral, and mortise views. A Canale view (15° pronation of the foot and the tube angled 75° cephalad) is useful to assess the talar profile.[33] The sensitivity of routine radiography is 50% to 75%. If there is still remaining concern after radiographs are normal, a bone scan can be useful as it is 99% sensitive.[30] However, MRI is typically the most common imaging tool used. An MRI is routinely indicated for diagnosis and preoperatively planning as it allows a good evaluation of the cartilage surface, underlying stability of the fragment, surrounding bony edema, and other soft tissue injuries. A CT scan is also often indicated to accurately assess lesion size, as MRI overestimates the size of the lesion secondary to bone edema.[30,34] CT will also assess for cystic or bony involvement. The correlation between the MRI imaging and arthroscopic findings is quite accurate, as MRI evaluations will coincide with the arthroscopic grading up to 81% to 83%.[35,36]

If a fresh allograft is planned, the patient's contralateral talus is used as a template and sized on CT. We attempt to match the size and shape of the allograft as closely as possible to the patient's native anatomy. Specifications are then sent to a tissue bank agency to obtain a whole talus of a matching size, but the final measurement is up to the surgeon. An allograft differing up to 2 mm from the native talus is considered acceptable. Osteochondral allografts should be obtained from US Food and Drug Administration (FDA)-approved suppliers who comply with the guidelines of the American Association of Tissue Banks. The donor talus is sterilely harvested within 24 hours of death. Next, the allograft undergoes disease testing and sterility culturing for approximately 2 weeks. During this time, the donor's medical history is reviewed for factors, such as high-risk behavior, that may lead to an unacceptable graft. The graft is maintained at 2 °C to 4 °C. If the graft passes, it is then processed and is shipped, usually within 3 weeks. The graft typically arrives at the hospital in 1 day. Surgical timing must be flexible to accommodate this process.

Surgical considerations of fresh talar allografts

First and foremost, a surgeon's approach is dictated by the location and size of the lesion. If one is planning a hemitalar allograft, the easiest approach is a standard anterior approach to the ankle. Access here is quite easy, with some planning. In fact, a significant portion of the talus can be accessed perpendicularly without a malleolar osteotomy. In a somewhat fortuitous turn of events, patients with these lesions often have ligamentous instability, which allows easier exposure from any surgical point of view. A perpendicular access allows the most control over cleanly resecting the diseased talus. The precision of sagittal and coronal talar cuts leaves more native talus, allows for reproducibility in recreating the dimensions to template our osteotomy in the fresh allograft talus, and grants a better reduction and fixation which can help decrease the rates of nonunion or subsidence. In a cadaveric study,[37] only 17% of the medial talar dome and 20% of the lateral talar dome could not be accessed without an osteotomy. After a lateral or medial malleolar osteotomy, the entire half of the talus could be accessed perpendicularly. After an anterolateral tibia osteotomy, there is an increase in sagittal exposure by 22%. Only the central 15% of the talar dome remains inaccessible perpendicularly. For smaller lesions (those that do not require half the talus to be resected) that are more posterior, the authors prefer to gain access to the joint via a malleolar osteotomy so that one may perpendicular access to the lesion.

Medial malleolar osteotomy

After marking out the centerline of the axis of the tibia and the anteromedial joint line, a 10-cm incision is made with 6 cm over the tibia and the remainder curved toward the navicular tubercle. At this point, two structures are important to protect: the posterior tibial tendon and saphenous vein. The periosteum is not to be breached except for the level of the osteotomy. To gain visualization of the lesion and the joint, a small capsulotomy is made anteromedially. At this point, one should have decided on the type of fixation for the osteotomy. The authors prefer two 4.0 cannulated screws (stainless steel or titanium is acceptable, but we prefer screws made of a biointegrative fiber-reinforced implant, Ossio, Woburn, MA) and an antiglide plate (one-third tubular plate). Although we perform an oblique osteotomy, a step cut (shaped like a chevron) is another stable construct.[37] Drill holes for the screws are then predrilled. Fluoroscopy is brought in and a 1.6-mm K-wire is drilled in the orientation of the osteotomy (**Fig. 1**). It is important to note that one needs to go slightly more beyond laterally since that will give the surgeon perpendicular access. The osteotomy should look more aggressive than one was planning.

Next, the posterior tibial tendon is protected posterior with a blunt Hohmann retractor. Fluoroscopy is then used to direct the cut. Before penetration into the joint, we use a half inch straight osteotome to complete the osteotomy. We then gently reflect the medial malleolus on the deltoid ligament, oftentimes needing to release the posterior capsular attachments. We then use a 2.0-mm K-wire to fixation the fragment.

Once the allograft transfer is complete, anatomic reduction of the joint is necessary. The kerf of the sawblade will make the osteotomy look slightly malreduced fluoroscopically, but the joint line should line up nicely. We then place our 2 4.0 mm screws followed by the four-hole one-third tubular plate in order to better fixate the osteotomy.

Lateral approach

A 10-cm incision is placed over the anterior fibula and centered over the joint line. We will first release the anterior talofibular ligament leaving a cuff of it to repair after surgery. Sometimes, the talus is mobile enough to obtain access to the lesion by drawing

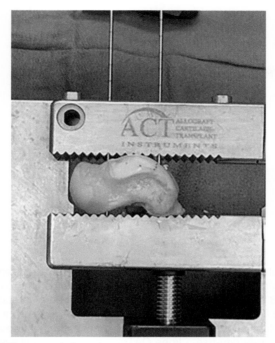

Fig. 1. Secure stabilization of the talus is important when harvesting the plug or block allograft.

it forward and rotating it plantarly, but more times than not, one must perform a fibular osteotomy. Subperiosteal dissection is completed around the fibula osteotomy site which is planned with fluoroscopy (the exit should be 1 cm proximal to the joint line). We use a microsagittal saw to create a long oblique osteotomy from superolateral to inferomedial. The osteotomy should be long enough to be reduced and fixated with two 3.5 mm lag screws. The syndesmotic ligaments are incised anteriorly and the fibula can be rotated posteriorly. Two 2.0 mm K-wires and a Hintermann distractor can aid with exposure.

Anterior approach

We place an incision 9 cm over the midline of the anterior ankle. The incision should be centered over one-third of the tibia and two-thirds of the talus. After we incise skin, we dissect down to the anterior retinacular layer, careful to avoid or identify and protect the superficial peroneal nerve. We make a small nick in the retinacular layer and then use Metzenbaum scissors to carefully release the exposed retinaculum. At this point, the tibialis anterior is exposed. We pull the tendon medially and incise sharply down to tibia, careful to avoid the neurovascular bundle. We then incise into the capsule, careful to respect the cartilage. Once the talus is exposed, we place two 1.6 mm K-wires under fluoroscopic guidance to guide our saw. With a perfect lateral view, the two views should appear as one and perpendicular to the sagittal axis of the joint (**Fig. 2**).

Circular Block Allograft

Anytime a talar allograft is used, we like to harvest autologous bone marrow aspirate concentrate (BMAC) from the anterior iliac crest to bath our allograft piece before

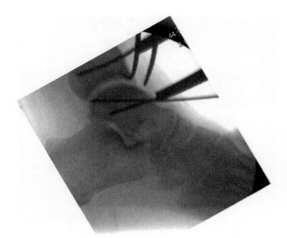

Fig. 2. Planning for the hemitalar allograft.

placement. One should understand the restraints of the allograft templating system one is using. Plug allografts should be reserved for contained, non-shoulder lesions. In the ankle OATS system (Arthrex, Naples, FL), the largest diameter of the lesion is 20 mm. Therefore, if one needs a larger plug, one may have to use a snowman technique of placing plugs sequentially next to each other such that it resembles a snowman. Alternatively, one can use a knee OATs system or musculoskeletal transplant foundation (MTF) (Miami, FL) set up for a larger circular plug. Each company has its own advantages and disadvantages, which will not be discussed here. Of note, certain companies offer precut Osteochondral cores at 10 mm or 16 mm sizes. These cores are not from the talus, however, rather the knee.

Once the osteochondral defect is visualized, a guide pin is drilled into the defect perpendicularly. A cannulated sizer is then placed over the lesion to determine its dimensions and chose an appropriate reamer. We will typically ream 10 to 12 mm deep to get to healthy bone. Once the reamer and guide pin are removed, the fresh talus allograft is secured to a holder (**Fig. 3**). The graduated donor harvester is then directed in the precise orientation such that the donor articular surface matches the recipient's. The donor talus is then drilled to the recipient's corresponding depth. The graft is extracted and thoroughly irrigated with saline. We then soak the allograft in BMAC for 5 minutes. One can dilate the recipient bed by 0.5 mm in order to better accommodate the donor plug, but we prefer a solid press fit. The allograft is then placed into the recipient site with gentle impaction.

Hemitalar allograft
Once we outline the osteotomy with the K-wires as described above, we then take a reciprocating saw to create a cut in the sagittal plane. Once that is complete, a sagittal saw (we use an 8 mm sawblade from a total ankle set). We then cut the recipient talus in the coronal plane under careful fluoroscopic guidance. The cut talar dome should be easily removed. Once this is removed, we measure carefully and draw these dimensions on the donor talus with a surgical skin marker. Here, it is important to match the precise angulation of one's cuts to not introduce inadvertent irregularities. We use a microsagittal saw and reciprocating saw blade after the talus is affixed to the donor holder. Once the donor talus allograft piece is removed, we again irrigate it thoroughly and then bathe it in BMAC. We then place the donor allograft into the recipient

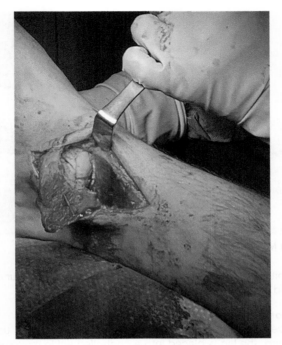

Fig. 3. At completion of the in situ osteotomy.

bed visualizing the contour matching as fluoroscopy is notoriously reliable. Once we are satisfied with placement, we then pin the talus with two 1.2 mm K-wires from medially or laterally to not disturb the cartilage. We then plantarflex the talus and place 2.0 mm lag screws across the osteotomy site, ensure that the cartilage is countersunk prior such that the metallic heads will not scuff the tibial cartilage. Fluoroscopic images at the point will be useful to ensure the appropriate length of the screws, but are deceiving when determining joint congruity. We then use fibrin glue to protect our osteotomy sites from joint fluid.

Small Rectangular Block Allograft

This method is useful when the lesion is a smaller shoulder lesion that is not amenable for OATS or too small to consider a hemitalar allograft. Here, inspecting the lesion perpendicularly allows one to cut out just enough talus to remove the diseased portion (**Fig. 4**). A combination of a microsagittal saw and reciprocating saw blade is useful. We remove a depth of roughly 8 to 10 mm depending on what our preoperative CT scan dictates. Once the diseased osteoarticular bone is removed, we measure and draw these dimensions on the donor talus with a surgical skin marker (**Figs. 5** and **6**). We use a microsagittal saw and reciprocating saw blade after the talus is secured. Once the donor talus allograft piece is removed, we again irrigate it thoroughly and then place it in BMAC. We then place the donor allograft into the recipient bed, visualizing the contour match. Once we are satisfied with placement, we then pin the talus to not damage the cartilage. Oftentimes, we place two 2.0 mm screws from medial to lateral (or lateral to medial) (**Figs. 7** and **8**). Often times, if we get a good press fit, we will use one screw or two chondral darts perpendicular to the osteotomy similar how

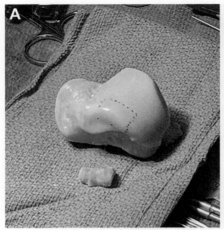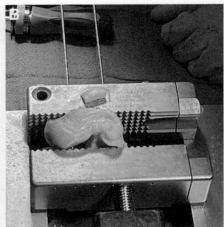

Fig. 4. (*A*) and (*B*) Measure twice and cut once.

we fixate the hemitalar allograft. We then use fibrin glue to protect our osteotomy sites from synovial fluid.

Postoperative protocol
Patients are placed into a non-weight-bearing splint for 2 weeks until stitches are removed. Afterward, the leg is placed into a controlled ankle movement (CAM) boot with strict non-weight-bearing precautions for 4 more weeks. At week 4 postoperatively, the patient is allowed to plantar and dorsiflex the ankle. At 6 weeks, the patient is allowed to walk in the boot once radiographs confirm early healing. Swimming and recumbent biking are allowed. Physical therapy focusing first on a range of motion and

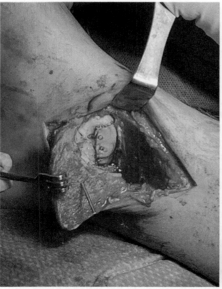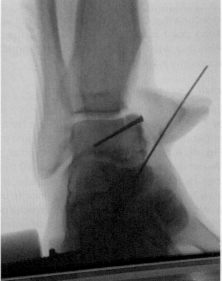

Fig. 5. Fixation of the medial talar allograft.

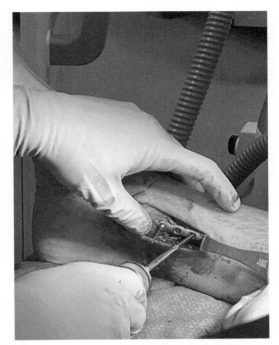

Fig. 6. Fixation of the medial malleolar osteotomy.

then strengthening is started, followed by proprioception. By week 10 to 12, the patient may walk in an athletic shoe. We do not allow high-impact exercise at least until 20 weeks from surgery.

Complications

Complications can occur at the host–host or graft–host interface, or be graft-mediated. Each has its own solutions, though oftentimes not satisfactory to either the surgeon or patient. Arthritis can still progress if the graft fails, or if there is an articular incongruity that alters joint mechanics. In a cadaver talar allograft study, flush graft placement restored near-normal contact pressures.[38] Malleolar osteotomies can sometimes fail to unite or be subject to malunion. In the case of nonunion, revision

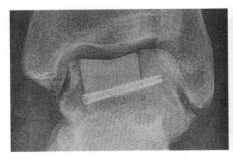
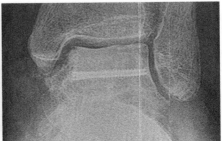

Fig. 7. x-ray of a structural allograft intraoperative and 8 months postoperative showing complete healing. (Photo included with permission from Dr David Dahlstrom.)

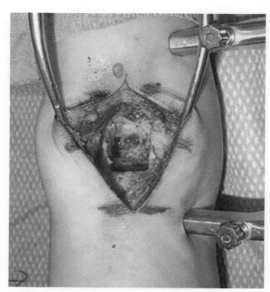

Fig. 8. Intraoperative photo showing exposure achieved with a mini anterior approach with a pin distractor. (Photo included with permission from Dr David Dahlstrom.)

open reduction and internal fixation with more robust implants is often needed. We will add autogenous bone graft to the construct as well. Sometimes, patients will complain of stiffness (arthrofibrosis). If physical therapy fails, we will use an external stretching device (Dynasplint, Severna Park, MD). If this fails, we will perform an arthroscopic lysis of adhesions and debridement, along with a manipulation under anesthesia. Rarely, the screws can back out slightly after the graft heals. It is important to compare immediate postoperative radiographs as the screws will always look prominent. An open approach is needed to remove the screws.

Over a period of 1 to 4 years, the allograft is slowly incorporated by creeping substitution.[39] During the revascularization of the allograft, the allograft bone is extremely vulnerable to collapse.[40] Failure most commonly occurs in the osseous portion of the graft, as this area can have subchondral collapse, delayed union, and nonunion with the recipient bone. The most common mechanisms of failure are graft fragmentation[41] and collapse and can manifest as new-onset pain, ankle swelling, and mechanical symptoms.[42] These grafts can have chondrolysis or cartilage delamination. Furthermore, these grafts may be subject to immune-mediated failure as a histopathologic analysis of eight retrieved, failed talar allografts demonstrated that graft failure seemed to be biologic.[43]

Revision options

Complications stemming from talar osteochondral allograft transfers can be quite high, but nothing is as devastating as graft failure. Failure has been reported as high as 35% in the literature.[44] Treatment options and their success rates are rarely reported or investigated. Common revision options include revision allograft transfer, bipolar allograft, three-dimensional printed total talus, ankle fusion, or ankle replacement. Although an ankle fusion may seem to be the most reliable revision option, often the failures occur in younger patients who would then suffer from adjacent hindfoot arthritis.[45] Total ankle replacement is an excellent option if there is not too much talar osteonecrosis or graft collapse to interfere with good bony ingrowth of the talar component. One might have to use a flat cut talar option because it will more reliably resect the collapsed portion of the talus.

A recent systematic review of allograft failure options examined a pool of 522 ankles in 11 studies.[46] The allograft failure rate was 11.5% with a reoperation rate of 18.9%. Reoperations included hardware removal, malunion open reduction internal fixation, revisions, and arthroscopic debridement. The weighted mean age was 30.3 years with a mean time to revision surgery of 53.3 months. Of the 84 reported revision cases, 30 (35.7%) were converted to a revision allograft, 20 (23.8%) were converted to total ankle replacement, and 34 (40.5%) were converted to ankle fusion. In a long-term follow-up of revision talar allograft procedures, Gaul and colleagues reported a 5- and 10-year survivorship of 84% and 65%, respectively.[47]

Outcomes

Literature involving fresh talar allograft transplantation consists of small case series without long-term follow-up. In a recent analysis of structural allograft transplantation at a mean follow-up of 56.2, Fletcher and colleagues examined 31 prospectively enrolled patients with a mean age of 41.4.[48] They found a relatively high graft survival rate of 96.8%. They noted that an MRI overestimates the mean lesion size on CT scan (3877 mm^3 vs 1879 mm^3). They noted significant improvements in visual analogue scale (VAS) score (20.3 at final follow-up), 36-item short form health survey (SF-36), and short musculoskeletal function assessment (SMFA) bother and function index at final follow-up. Fifteen (48.4%) patients underwent an additional surgery, most commonly arthroscopic debridement or removal of hardware. There was one failure that then underwent a total ankle replacement.

Raikin[49] reviewed 15 cases of fresh block-shaped allografts of the talus. At a mean follow-up of 44 months, the evidence of collapse or resorption of the graft was seen radiographically in 66% of 10 patients. In addition, 60% demonstrated some narrowing of the joint space overlying the graft area. Hahn and colleagues reviewed 13 patients with a block-shaped allograft at a mean of 48 months follow-up.[50] All the patients were all satisfied with the results, but 12/13 patients developed osteophytes and other mild arthritic changes were seen in two patients. Haene and colleagues reported prospectively the results of 17 block-shaped allografts at a mean follow-up of 4.1 years.[51] Five ankles were considered failures (29.4%), whereas two had poor, six good, and four excellent results.

A recent systematic review conducted by Migliorini and colleagues reviewed from 40 studies (1174 procedures) with a mean follow-up of 46.5 months with an intent to compare autograft versus allograft transplantation.[52] The magnetic resonance observation of cartilage repair tissue (MOCART) and American Orthopaedic Foot & Ankle Society (AOFAS) scores were better in the autograft group, whereas the VAS score was similar between the two groups (2.4). Interestingly, autografts demonstrated a lower rate of revision surgery (10.2% vs 44.9%; OR, 7.2) and failure (3.3% vs 14.7%; OR, 5.1).

CLINICS CARE POINTS

- First and foremost, a surgeon's approach is dictated by the location and size of the lesion. If one is planning a hemitalar allograft, the easiest approach is a standard anterior approach to the ankle.

- Cartilage viability is required for successful clinical outcomes after transplantation of osteochondral allografts, so storage and handling are very important.

- Generally, osteochondral allograft transplantation is not first-line treatment unless the lesion is large (>1.5 cm) or a shoulder lesion as allograft can be shaped to address different locations and different lesion sizes.
- Preoperative planning includes obtaining x-rays, a CT scan, an MRI, and a single photon emission computed tomography (SPECT-CT) scan to define the location, size, cartilage surface, and joint condition.
- If a fresh allograft is planned, the patient's contralateral talus is used as a template and sized on CT. We attempt to match the size and shape of the allograft as closely as possible to the patient's native anatomy.

DISCLOSURE

The authors have no disclosures related to this worl.

REFERENCES

1. Leontaritis N, Hiˆ$nojosa L, Panchbhavi VK. Arthroscopically detected intra-articular lesions associated with acute ankle fractures. J Bone Joint Surg Am 2009;91(2):333–9.
2. Saxena A, Eakin C. Articular talar injuries in athletes: results of microfracture and autogenous bone graft. Am J Sports Med 2007;35(10):1680–7.
3. Tol JL, Struijs PA, Bossuyt PM, et al. Treatment strategies in osteochondral defects of the talar dome: a systematic review. Foot Ankle Int 2000;21(2):119–26.
4. Hintermann B, Regazzoni P, Lampert C, et al. Arthroscopic findings in acute fractures of the ankle. J Bone Joint Surg Br 2000;82(3):345–51.
5. Looze CA, Capo J, Ryan MK, et al. Evaluation and Management of Osteochondral Lesions of the Talus. Cartilage 2017;8(1):19–30.
6. Chu CH, Chen IH, Yang KC, et al. Midterm Results of Fresh-Frozen Osteochondral Allografting for Osteochondral Lesions of the Talus. Foot Ankle Int 2021; 42(1):8–16.
7. Zengerink M, Struijs PA, Tol JL, et al. Treatment of osteochondral lesions of the talus: a systematic review. Knee Surg Sports Traumatol Arthrosc 2010;18(2): 238–46.
8. Klammer G, Maquieira GJ, Spahn S, et al. Natural history of nonoperatively treated osteochondral lesions of the talus. Foot Ankle Int 2015;36(1):24–31.
9. O'Loughlin PF, Heyworth BE, Kennedy JG. Current concepts in the diagnosis and treatment of osteochondral lesions of the ankle. Am J Sports Med 2010;38(2): 392–404.
10. Powers RT, Dowd TC, Giza E. Surgical Treatment for Osteochondral Lesions of the Talus. Arthroscopy 2021;37(12):3393–6.
11. Hannon CP, Smyth NA, Murawski CD, et al. Osteochondral lesions of the talus: aspects of current management. Bone Joint Lett J 2014;96-B(2):164–71.
12. Gross CE, Adams SB, Easley ME, et al. Role of Fresh Osteochondral Allografts for Large Talar Osteochondral Lesions. J Am Acad Orthop Surg 2016;24(1):e9–17.
13. Shapiro F, Koide S, Glimcher MJ. Cell origin and differentiation in the repair of full-thickness defects of articular cartilage. J Bone Joint Surg Am 1993;75(4):532–53.
14. Murawski CDKJ. Prolongation of T2 stratification after microfracture does not indicate normal cartilage. Cartilage 2011;2(4):399.
15. Murawski CD, Foo LF, Kennedy JG. A Review of Arthroscopic Bone Marrow Stimulation Techniques of the Talus: The Good, the Bad, and the Causes for Concern. Cartilage 2010;1(2):137–44.

16. Mercer NPSA, Dankert JF, Kennedy JG. Outcomes of Autologous Osteochondral Transplantation With and Without Extracellular Matrix Cartilage Allograft Augmentation for Osteochondral Lesions of the Talus. Am J Sports Med 2022;50(1): 161–9. Epub 2021.

17. Smyth NA, Murawski CD, Haleem AM, et al. Establishing proof of concept: Platelet-rich plasma and bone marrow aspirate concentrate may improve cartilage repair following surgical treatment for osteochondral lesions of the talus. World J Orthop 2012;3(7):101–8.

18. Gianakos AL, Kennedy JG. Rethinking Cartilage Lesions of the Ankle: An Update on the Role of Biologic Adjuvants. J Am Acad Orthop Surg 2023. https://doi.org/10.5435/JAAOS-D-22-01042.

19. Hogan MV, Hicks JJ, Chambers MC, et al. Biologic Adjuvants for the Management of Osteochondral Lesions of the Talus. J Am Acad Orthop Surg 2019; 27(3):e105–11.

20. Zhu Y, Xu X. Osteochondral Autograft Transfer Combined With Cancellous Allografts for Large Cystic Osteochondral Defect of the Talus. Foot Ankle Int 2016; 37(10):1113–8.

21. Danilkowicz RM, Allen NB, Grimm N, et al. Histological and Inflammatory Cytokine Analysis of Osteochondral Lesions of the Talus After Failed Microfracture: Comparison With Fresh Allograft Controls. Orthop J Sports Med 2021;9(10). 23259671211040535.

22. Vogel J, Soti V. Effectiveness of Autograft and Allograft Transplants in Treating Athletic Patients With Osteochondral Lesions of the Talus. Cureus 2022;14(10): e29913.

23. Bisicchia S, Rosso F, Amendola A. Osteochondral allograft of the talus. Iowa Orthop J 2014;34:30–7.

24. Williams SK, Amiel D, Ball ST, et al. Prolonged storage effects on the articular cartilage of fresh human osteochondral allografts. J Bone Joint Surg Am 2003; 85(11):2111–20.

25. Paul KD, Patel RK, Arguello AM, et al. Variability in the Processing of Fresh Osteochondral Allografts. J Knee Surg 2023;36(4):450–5.

26. Ranawat ASVA, Chen CT, Zelken JA, et al. Williams RJ Material properties of fresh cold-stored allografts for osteochondral defects at 1 year. Clin Orthop Relat Res 2008;466(8):1826–36.

27. Convery FR, Akeson WH, Amiel D, et al. Long-term survival of chondrocytes in an osteochondral articular cartilage allograft. A case report. J Bone Joint Surg Am 1996;78(7):1082–8.

28. Enneking WF, Campanacci DA. Retrieved human allografts: a clinicopathological study. J Bone Joint Surg Am 2001;83(7):971–86.

29. Enneking WF, Mindell ER. Observations on massive retrieved human allografts. J Bone Joint Surg Am 1991;73(8):1123–42.

30. Amendola A, Panarella L. Osteochondral lesions: medial versus lateral, persistent pain, cartilage restoration options and indications. Foot Ankle Clin 2009;14(2): 215–27.

31. Bauer M, Jonsson K, Linden B. Osteochondritis dissecans of the ankle. A 20-year follow-up study. J Bone Joint Surg Br 1987;69(1):93–6.

32. Pettine KA, Morrey BF. Osteochondral fractures of the talus. A long-term follow-up. J Bone Joint Surg Br 1987;69(1):89–92.

33. Canale ST, Kelly FB Jr. Fractures of the neck of the talus. Long-term evaluation of seventy-one cases. J Bone Joint Surg Am 1978;60(2):143–56.

34. Gortz S, De Young AJ, Bugbee WD. Fresh osteochondral allografting for osteochondral lesions of the talus. Foot Ankle Int 2010;31(4):283–90.
35. Lee KB, Bai LB, Park JG, et al. A comparison of arthroscopic and MRI findings in staging of osteochondral lesions of the talus. Knee Surg Sports Traumatol Arthrosc 2008;16(11):1047–51.
36. Mintz DN, Tashjian GS, Connell DA, et al. Osteochondral lesions of the talus: a new magnetic resonance grading system with arthroscopic correlation. Arthroscopy 2003;19(4):353–9.
37. Adams SB Jr, Demetracopoulos CA, Queen RM, et al. Early to mid-term results of fixed-bearing total ankle arthroplasty with a modular intramedullary tibial component. J Bone Joint Surg Am 2014;96(23):1983–9.
38. Latt LD, Glisson RR, Montijo HE, et al. Effect of graft height mismatch on contact pressures with osteochondral grafting of the talus. Am J Sports Med 2011;39(12):2662–9.
39. McDermott AG, Langer F, Pritzker KP, et al. Fresh small-fragment osteochondral allografts. Long-term follow-up study on first 100 cases. Clin Orthop Relat Res 1985;(197):96–102.
40. Meehan R, McFarlin S, Bugbee W, et al. Fresh ankle osteochondral allograft transplantation for tibiotalar joint arthritis. Foot Ankle Int 2005;26(10):793–802.
41. Juels CA, So E, Seidenstricker C, et al. Complications of En Bloc Osteochondral Talar Allografts and Treatment of Failures: Literature Review and Case Report. J Foot Ankle Surg 2020;59(1):149–55.
42. Okeagu CN, Baker EA, Barreras NA, et al. Review of Mechanical, Processing, and Immunologic Factors Associated With Outcomes of Fresh Osteochondral Allograft Transplantation of the Talus. Foot Ankle Int 2017;38(7):808–19.
43. Pomajzl RJ, Baker EA, Baker KC, et al. Case Series With Histopathologic and Radiographic Analyses Following Failure of Fresh Osteochondral Allografts of the Talus. Foot Ankle Int 2016;37(9):958–67.
44. Gross AE, Agnidis Z, Hutchison CR. Osteochondral defects of the talus treated with fresh osteochondral allograft transplantation. Foot Ankle Int 2001;22(5):385–91.
45. Coester LM, Saltzman CL, Leupold J, et al. Long-term results following ankle arthrodesis for post-traumatic arthritis. J Bone Joint Surg Am 2001;83(2):219–28.
46. Juels CA, So E, Seidenstricker C, et al. A Comparison of Outcomes of Revision Surgical Options for the Treatment of Failed Bulk Talar Allograft Transfer: A Systematic Review. J Foot Ankle Surg 2020;59(6):1265–71.
47. Gaul F, Tirico LEP, McCauley JC, et al. Long-term Follow-up of Revision Osteochondral Allograft Transplantation of the Ankle. Foot Ankle Int 2018;39(5):522–9.
48. Fletcher AN, Johnson LG, Easley ME, et al. Midterm Prospective Evaluation of Structural Allograft Transplantation for Osteochondral Lesions of the Talar Shoulder. Foot Ankle Int 2022;43(7):899–912.
49. Raikin SM. Fresh osteochondral allografts for large-volume cystic osteochondral defects of the talus. J Bone Joint Surg Am 2009;91(12):2818–26.
50. Hahn DB, Aanstoos ME, Wilkins RM. Osteochondral lesions of the talus treated with fresh talar allografts. Foot Ankle Int 2010;31(4):277–82.
51. Haene R, Qamirani E, Story RA, et al. Intermediate outcomes of fresh talar osteochondral allografts for treatment of large osteochondral lesions of the talus. J Bone Joint Surg Am 2012;94(12):1105–10.
52. Migliorini F, Maffulli N, Baroncini A, et al. Allograft Versus Autograft Osteochondral Transplant for Chondral Defects of the Talus: Systematic Review and Meta-analysis. Am J Sports Med 2022;50(12):3447–55.

Cartilage Injuries
Basic Science Update

Albert T. Anastasio, MD, Samuel B. Adams, MD*

KEYWORDS

- Chondral injury • OCD • Osteochondral lesions • Basic science • Cartilage lesions
- Microfracture • Bone marrow stimulation • ACI

KEY POINTS

- Proinflammatory cytokines and matrix metalloproteinases play a key role in mediation of the onset of posttraumatic arthritis after an ankle injury.
- Bone marrow stimulation is a reasonably effective treatment of chondral injuries, and various means to enhance outcomes after stimulation procedures have been developed and are currently being studied.
- Genetic modulation of mesenchymal stem cells is an ongoing area of substantial research, and novel therapeutics will be designed within the next several decades, which have the potential to revolutionize care for foot and ankle pathologic condition.

INTRODUCTION

Articular cartilage is a highly specialized connective tissue consisting of extracellular matrix (ECM) components, including chondrocytes, collagen fibers (predominantly type II and type IX), small noncollagen proteins (such as aggrecan, high molecular weight proteoglycan, and cartilage oligomeric matrix protein), water, and a small volume of glycoproteins such as fibronectin.[1] This biomolecular make-up is highly regulated by chondrocytes in response to their environmental changes, exhibiting profound capacity to modulate activity based on chemical and mechanical signals.[2]

The articular cartilage of the foot and ankle differs from the cartilage of the other joints of the lower extremity. Ankle cartilage is stiffer and has less permeability than the cartilage of the knee due to a higher water and protein glycogen content.[3] It is also thinner than the articular cartilage of the knee (1–1.62 mm vs 1.69–2.55 mm).[3] It has a dense ECM, which is thought to improve load-bearing capacity and reduce the susceptibility of the joint to mechanical damage.[4] Chondrocytes found within the ankle joint have been demonstrated to exhibit more metabolic activity than the

Division of Foot and Ankle Surgery, Department of Orthopaedic Surgery, Duke University Health System, 311 Trent Drive, Durham, NC 27710, USA
* Corresponding author. Department of Orthopaedic Surgery, Duke University Medical Center, 5601 Arringdon Park Drive, Suite 300, Morrisville, NC 27560.
E-mail address: samuel.adams@duke.edu

Foot Ankle Clin N Am 29 (2024) 357–369
https://doi.org/10.1016/j.fcl.2023.08.002
1083-7515/24/© 2023 Elsevier Inc. All rights reserved.

foot.theclinics.com

chondrocytes of the knee, eliciting a greater response to anabolic factors such as osteogenic protein-1 and C-propeptide of type II collagen.[5] They demonstrate less sensitivity to catabolic signaling mechanisms such as fibronectin and interleukin (IL)-1 beta.[5] These factors serve to improve the restorative capacity of ankle cartilage.

Despite the remarkable ability of ankle cartilage to self-regenerate, high rates of posttraumatic arthritis of the ankle are encountered after ligamentous and bony injuries. Investigation during the last few decades has substantially improved our understanding of the complex posttraumatic milieu that contributes to the rapid progression of arthritis in the ankle.[6] Proinflammatory cytokines (eg, *IL-1β*, *tumor necrosis factor [TNF]-α*, *IL-6*, *IL-15*, *IL-17*, and *IL-18*), metalloproteinases (MMPs; adamalysins, disintegrin, and *ADAMs*), aberrancies in growth factors (fibroblast growth factor [*FGF*] and transforming growth factor [*TGF*]-*β*), and immunologic adaptations (major histocompatibility system [MHC] class I complex formation and MHC class II and *ICAM*-1 intercellular adhesion molecule upregulation) all are thought to lead to onset of posttraumatic arthritis.[7]

As our understanding of the complex processes that govern articular cartilage increases, targeted therapies are being developed that may support that innate ability of the ankle to regenerate damaged cartilage. The purpose of this review, therefore, is to explore new developments in the basic science research pertaining to cartilage, with an emphasis on points of relevance to the foot and ankle surgeon. We will explore new advances in investigation of the biomolecular contributors to the inflammatory milieu, which is thought to contribute to cartilage degradation, genetic and epigenetic changes that underwrite arthritis, and translational advancements within the therapeutics used to target chondral damage in the foot and ankle.

BASIC SCIENCE OF CARTILAGE INJURY

The inflammatory milieu, which ultimately leads to cartilage injury and the onset of posttraumatic arthritis is remarkably complex, and our knowledge regarding this environment increases yearly as new signaling factors and biomolecular pathways are discovered. Categorization of the contributors to the posttraumatic milieu can prove difficult because a complex interplay governs the interaction between various chemical and cellular substrates. For the purposes of this review, 4 categories will be explored relating to the posttraumatic milieu of the ankle to discuss recent advancements within the study of (1) MMPs, (2) growth factors, (3) inflammatory factors, and (4) genetic and epigenetic changes (**Fig. 1**).

Metalloproteinases

MMPs target the destruction of type II collagen and result in the irreversible proteolytic destruction of cartilage. There are 7 matrix MMPs, which are expressed in articular cartilage, and among these, only MMP-1, MMP-2, MMP-13, and MMP-14 are constitutively expressed in adult cartilage.[8] Thus, the presence of MMP-3, MMP-8, and MMP-9 seems to indicate an underlying pathologic process.[9] Notably, MMP-1, MMP-8, and MMP-13 are soluble and seem to contribute substantially to cartilage degradation.[10] MMP expression is regulated by several intracellular signaling pathways: proinflammatory and pleiotropic cytokines and growth factors have been found to govern the action of MMP.[11] Moreover, there is a strong positive relationship between the rate of joint destruction and the increase in MMP expression.[12–15]

Several important findings relating to MMPs have surfaced in recent years. MMP-13, as 1 of the only 3 soluble MMPs, is capable of triple-helical collagen cleavage and demonstrates a strong preference for type II collagen.[16] Given the profound

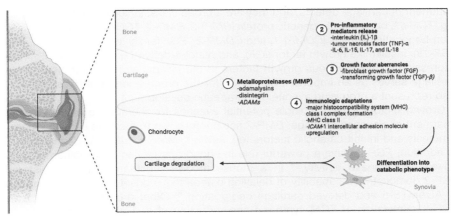

Fig. 1. The role of the 4 major mediators of cartilage degradation: (1) metalloproteinases (adamalysins, disintegrin, and *ADAMs*), (2) proinflammatory cytokines (eg, *IL-1β, TNF-α, IL-6, IL-15, IL-17,* and *IL-18*), (3) aberrancies in growth factors (*FGF* and *TGF-β*), and (4) immunologic adaptations (major histocompatibility system [MHC]) class I complex formation and MHC class II and *ICAM-1* intercellular adhesion molecule upregulation.

role of this compound in cartilage degradation, MMP-13 has been the subject of much investigation in recent years. In better characterizing MMP-13 and its relationships, crystal structures have revealed the mode of binding for MMP-1, a related collagenase, which acts in concert with MMP-13.[17] Moreover, catalytic and hemopexin domains have been shown to play several essential roles in this interaction.[18] Several molecules have been found to serve as activators of MMP-13, including plasmin[19] and other MMPs such as MMP-14.[20] In addition, an increase in MMP-13 activity in cultures treated with activated protein C was demonstrated in human osteoarthritic cartilage chondrocytes.[21] Further characterization of MMP-13 binding sites in addition to the identification of novel downregulatory molecules of this MMP may lead to the development of targeted therapies for the treatment of arthritis.

Intuitively, a greater appreciation of the major endogenous inhibitors for cartilage degradatory MMPs may lead to powerful therapeutics with direct repressive effects on MMP degradative activity. Four members of tissue inhibitors of metalloproteases (TIMPs) are expressed in human tissues. Each TIMP exhibits a 2-domain structure consisting of an N-terminal domain (comprising a "wedge-shaped" ridge, which binds to the MMP active site) and a C-terminal domain (responsible for interacting with the hemopexin domain).[22] Each of the 4 human TIMPs has been the subject of ongoing investigation but TIMP-3 in particular exhibits a chondroprotective role in cartilage. Increased cartilage collagen damage has been demonstrated in aged mice deficient in TIMP-3.[23] Contributing to their potential as a therapeutic agent, TIMPs can be structurally engineered. Mutants of TIMP-3, which selectively inhibit a disintegrin and MMP with thrombospondin motifs 4 (A disintegrin and metalloproteinase with thrombospondin motifs [ADAMTS]-4) and ADAMTS-5 have been constructed.[24] Advances in TIMP engineering such as these may improve selectivity for particular MMPs and allow for powerful modulation of the inflammatory milieu within synovial fluid.

Growth Factors

Growth factors within cartilage serve as enhancers of chondrogenesis and stimulators of cell growth. They constitute biologically active polypeptides that can support the treatment of cartilage defects, and they are a broad class, including *TGF* superfamily (eg, *TGF-β1*, bone morphogenetic protein [*BMP*]-2, *BMP-7*, *TGF-β3*, *cartilage*-derived morphogenetic proteins [*CDMP*]-1, and *CDMP-2*), *FGF* family (eg, *bFGF*, *FGF-2*, and *FGF-18*), insulin-like growth factor (*IGF*), and platelet-derived growth factor.[25–27] The expression of these various growth factors in the inflammatory environment within cartilage serves as an important biomarker for the progression of arthritis and may also represent a promising avenue of therapeutic development.

Growth factors exhibit multiple potential avenues for therapeutic efficacy in the treatment of diseased cartilage. *BMP-7* has been shown to promote cartilage matrix synthesis and inhibit catabolic factors (eg, *MMP-1*, *MMP-13*, *IL-1*, *IL-6*, and *IL-8*).[28] In addition, *FGF-2* plays a powerful role in chondroprotection by inhibition of IL-1-driven aggrecanase activity.[29] In a mouse model, subcutaneously administered FGF-2 demonstrates capability of delaying osteoarthritis onset through suppression of ADAMTS-5 and delayed cartilage degradation.[30] Other growth factors such as *TGF-β* (stimulation of ECM synthesis and reduction of *IL-1* catabolic activity) and IGF-1 (promotion of synovial membrane protection) have demonstrated chondroprotective effects and serve as potential target for therapeutic application.[31]

Inflammatory Factors

A large number of factors correlating with the inflammatory cascade have been shown to contribute to the onset of cartilage destruction and osteoarthritis. A growing body of research outlines these cytokines and their contribution to joint disease. The inflammatory factors associated with arthritis can be grouped as follows: (1) inflammatory mediators (cyclooxygenase, prostaglandin E2, *PGD2*, *PGF2a*, *PGI2*, and thromboxane); (2) circulating or locally occurring cytokines: *IL-1*, *IL-6*, *IL-17*, *IL-18*, *TNF-α*, and chemokines, such as C-C motif chemokine ligand 5 and *IL-8*; (3) nitric oxide (NO); and (4) synovial degradation products including hyaluronan or hyaluronic acid.[32]

Other proinflammatory mediators that are less intimately linked with arthritic conditions but have nonetheless demonstrated elevations in joint-diseased states include vascular endothelial growth factor (*VEGF*), blood vessel formation (factor VIII), intercellular adhesion molecule-1, and other proinflammatory cytokines (*TNF-α*, *IL-6*, and *IL-1β*).[33] The relationship of these various moieties with cartilage degradation is complex, and proposed mechanisms include the overexpression of MMP, the paracrine stimulation of cellular release of other proinflammatory cytokines and growth factors, the induction of chondrocyte apoptosis, the inhibition of glycoprotein and collagen synthesis, and the stimulation of NO production.[34] Thus, therapeutics targeting the inflammatory cascade may have far-reaching and potent efficacy.

Genetic and Epigenetic Changes

Profound advancement in our capacity to understand and modulate the complex genetic and epigenetic environment of the osteoarthritic joint has occurred during the last several decades. Tong and colleagues established the relationship of 2 common allelic variants of *MMP-3* (*rs650108*) and *TIMP-3* (*rs715572*) with the risk of onset of arthritis.[35] Metanalysis from Wang and colleagues reviewed 56 single nucleotide polymorphisms (SNPs) from different genes that have been shown to be associated with osteoarthritis (OA), including SNPs in *COL11A1*, *TGF-1β*, *VEGF*, *IL-6*, *ASPN*, *GDF5*, *CALM1*, and *SMAD3*.[36] With regards to areas of potential therapeutic application, SNPs in the *MMP-3* gene have experimentally demonstrated a contribution to an increased risk of arthritis and may serve as biomarkers for susceptibility to the condition.[37] Moreover, substantial study has centered on the effect of *GDF5*, a prominent genetic risk factor associated with OA. The rs143383 SNP has been shown to significantly reduce the transcriptional activity of GDF5 in chondrocytes, resulting in maintenance by resident cells and the disruption of cartilage synthesis.[38] Through regulating GDF5 activity, drug developers hope to influence the healing of connective tissue and reduce the onset of arthritis. Indeed, Parrish and colleagues demonstrated a significant reduction in disease progression in osteoarthritic joints after intra-articular supplementation of recombinant human GDF5.[39]

Epigenetic factors also influence the progression of arthritis, with special attention given to microRNAs in recent years. These low molecular weight, noncoding RNAs can already be used as predictors of disease and may have potential far beyond diagnostic purposes. MicroRNAs are posttranscriptional regulators of gene expression and may be an ideal candidate for personalized therapy.[40] Modulation of microRNA activity may profoundly influence the inflammatory cascade, leading to multiple downstream ramifications that ultimately can lead to chondroprotection.[41] At the cutting edge of pharmaceutical innovation, various delivery mechanisms including nanomaterial constructions have been tested in vivo and hold great promise for the future treatment and prevention of arthritis.[42–44]

Therapeutics for Cartilage Injury

As our understanding of the biomolecular pathways of cartilage degradation grows, so does our capacity to modulate the inflammatory environment, slow the progression of disease, and in some cases, reverse symptoms of arthritis. A comprehensive review of recent advancements in the translational science of cartilage regeneration would be impossible given space limitations, and the goal of this review will be to discuss several recent developments and avenues for potential therapeutic efficacy to inform the foot and ankle surgeon interested in new directions in cartilage repair. An emphasis will be placed on literature directly related to foot and ankle but animal cartilage models involving other joints will also be discussed.

Marrow Stimulation

Marrow stimulation techniques such as lesion debridement and microfracture have been extensively studied for osteochondral lesions of the talus (OLT), with varying degrees of efficacy.[45–49] Novel advancements within the domain of marrow stimulation may improve the natural cartilage repair mechanisms and improve patient outcomes, although many of these developments remain in the early phases of investigation. Ivkovic and colleagues assessed the utility of ovine autologous bone marrow transduced with adenoviral vectors containing cDNA for green fluorescent protein or TGF (TGF-β1) and formulated into a plug for implantation on partial-thickness medial condylar defects in a sheep model.[50] The TGF-treated condylar defects showed significantly greater amounts of collagen II deposition. FGF-2 and IGF-1 have also been delivered by a transgene conduit in rabbit osteochondral defect model and have demonstrated favorable results.[51,52]

Several gene-based techniques have also been used to enhance marrow stimulation. Pascher and colleagues targeted bone marrow-derived cells for genetic modification in an effort to enhance natural cartilage repair mechanisms. These authors demonstrated the feasibility of mixing an adenoviral suspension with the fluid phase of freshly aspirated bone marrow to result in uniform vector dispersion throughout the collected sample. They determined a directly proportional rate of transgenic expression to the density of nucleated cells in the corresponding clot.[53] This study allows for targeted gene delivery to cartilage defects. Other authors have applied this method, including Sieker and colleagues who used using cDNA that encoded

BMP-2 and Indian hedgehog protein to improve cartilage repair in osteochondral defects in the trochlea of rabbit knees.[54]

At this time, there is a paucity of clinical studies on the use of specific growth factors to supplement marrow stimulation. However, several studies have added various orthobiologic products to marrow stimulation, including bone marrow aspirate concentrate (BMAC) and platelet rich plasma (PRP). These products contain substantial quantities of growth factors and other bimolecularly active compounds. Murphey and colleagues compared 52 patients with OLT receiving microfracture alone to 49 patients receiving microfracture plus BMAC. Both groups had improvements in pain scores, quality of life scores, and degree of participation in sport but the revision rate was statistically significantly lower (12.2%) in the microfracture plus BMAC group versus the microfracture alone group (28.8%).[55] Botta and colleagues included 7 studies in a meta-analysis evaluating the addition of PRP to microfracture in osteochondral defects of the knee and ankle. Although improvements were noted with the addition of PRP, the improvement offered by PRP did not reach the minimal clinically important difference value required to recommend the widespread use of the PRP in all cases of microfracture, especially given the extensive cost of the product.[56]

Autologous Chondrocyte Implantation

Autologous chondrocyte implantation (ACI), including matrix autologous chondrocyte implantation (MACI), has shown promise in the treatment of osteochondral defects, including OLT.[57–60] Although multiple methodologies have been approved for ACI, all procedures involve 2 surgical stages. First, articular cartilage is harvested from a non–weight-bearing or lesser weight-bearing donor site and subsequently expanded in culture under various growth conditions. A second-stage procedure involves implantation of the cultured cells into the cartilage defect. As with marrow stimulation techniques, several adjuncts have been used with ACI with demonstrated efficacy. For example, Richter and colleagues report the outcomes of 129 patients with 136 chondral lesions of the ankle treated with MACI plus peripheral blood concentrate. Average lesion size was 1.8 cm^2. Improvements in pain scores and functional outcomes were noted at both the 2-year and 5-year follow-up time points.[61]

Although shown to be efficacious, ACI is expensive and requires substantial resources given the necessity for the staged approach. Thus, the use of genetically modified allografted chondrocytes has been proposed as a cost-saving alternative to ACI. The use of genetically modified allografted chondrocytes is backed by a growing body of animal research, which confirms efficacy in cartilage repair and an excellent safety profile.[62] These chondrocytes have been shown to persist and express transgenes in rabbit osteochondral defects.[63] Through transference of various growth factors and mediators of cartilage repair, both autograft and allograft chondrocytes can be primed for greater potency in vivo. Ortved and colleagues demonstrated the capacity for improved repair of full-thickness chondral defects in equines treated with autologous chondrocytes with transduced *IGF-1*.[64] These methodologies could be applied to allograft chondrocytes by similar means.

This technology has progressed to the extent whereby genetically enhanced allograft chondrocytes have been used in human clinical trials. Using a line of chondrocytes obtained from a newborn with polydactyly, Ha and colleagues surgically introduced cells into cartilage lesions using a fibrin scaffold. A retrovirus carrying *TGF-β1* cDNA was transduced into one of the cellular expansions, and results trended toward improved outcomes in the patients receiving this particular cell line. The study was inadequately powered to note statistically significant improvements in the group receiving allograft exposed to retrovirus-transduced *TGF-β1* cDNA but these promising results lend credence to the assertion that allograft-derived products can be enhanced through the use of genetic modification.[65]

Muscle/Fat Grafts and Scaffolds

Skeletal muscle and fat contain an abundance of cellular products and growth factors that, if chemically or mechanically altered and applied to an appropriate scaffold or delivery mechanism, could yield cartilage-regenerative properties. Moreover, these processes can be truncated into a time frame appropriate for single-stage procedures. For example, genetically modified, autologous skeletal muscle and fat grafts can be harvested and altered before being press-fit into an osteochondral lesion during a single surgical window. Skeletal muscle in particular contains satellite cells capable of forming postmitotic, multinucleated myotubes and myofibers, which can secrete growth factors and other morphogenetic moieties while additionally providing tissue-innate scaffolding properties. The skeletal muscle and fat grafts can be modulated through the use of, for example, adenovirus vectors carrying BMP2 cDNA, yielding bone deposition in subchondral region and cartilage above a bony defect in a rabbit model.[66]

Skeletal muscle and fat grafts demonstrate innate potential to act as a scaffold given their specific physical composition. However, the treatment of focal cartilage defects with other approaches lacking an appropriate scaffold can result in failure of delivery of cellular components, gene vectors, and chondroregenerative growth factors to the target site and dilution into synovial fluid.[67] Thus, various biomaterials have been developed for use as scaffolds for delivery of cartilage-targeting therapeutics. As the scaffold degrades over time, the contents contained within are slowly released to the target area, prolonging the duration of action. A scaffold also serves to prevent degradation of the therapeutic contents and allows for direct surgical visualization of lesion coverage confirming appropriate delivery.[68]

A vast diversity of synthetic derivatives has been developed for use as a scaffold material. In-depth discussion of each is beyond the scope of this article but the use of scaffolds for osteochondral tissue repair is generally carried out through 1 of 2 methods: (1) through incorporation of a viral gene vector with transferred genes encoding chondroprotective transcription factors during scaffold manufacturing and subsequently implanting this construct in a cartilage defect to transfect chondrocytes and promote healing or (2) through the connection of a formed scaffold directly with a vector with cells. Ideal scaffold materials are biocompatible and biodegradable and include several compounds such as self-assembling RAD16-I peptide hydrogels,[69] polymeric micelles,[70] and polypseudorotaxane gels[71] through a recombinant adeno-associated virus vector, and poly-e-caprolactone through a lentiviral vector.[72] Ongoing innovation will further define ideal scaffold materials and viral vectors for delivery of cartilage-regenerative moieties to damaged articular surfaces.

Mesenchymal Stem Cells

Although most of the previously discussed topics focus on delivery of various chemokines and growth factors to existing chondrocytes or direct application of modified autologous or allograft-derived chondrocytes to a cartilage defect, use of progenitor cells for the treatment of chondral loss is also a promising avenue for arthritis prevention and cartilage repair. Of the various forms of predifferentiated progenitor cells, mesenchymal stem cells (MSCs) are the most widely studied given their high capacity for proliferation, broad differentiation ability, and wide availability. Both adipose-derived MSCs and bone marrow-derived MSCs (BMSCs)[73] and adipose-derived MSCs (ASCs)[74] have been harvested for use in osteochondral injury. For example, Chimutenwende-Gordon and colleagues describe a technique for BMSC transplantation into osteochondral defects of the knee. They report success in a small sample of 3 patients.[75] Similarly, Freitag and colleagues applied ASCs to a large nonhealing osteochondral defect in the knee of a patient who had failed prior surgery, resulting in structural and functional improvement. Despite some promising early results, these technologies lack large sample-size studies with long-term follow-up.

MSCs can be concentrated within a sample and directly applied to a cartilage lesion with demonstrated efficacy in multiple in vivo models. However, in recent years, more emphasis has been placed on experimental models of augmented or genetically modified MSCs with the goal of creating amplified MSCs with more potent cartilage-repair potential. Three-dimensional fibrin–polyurethane scaffolds in a hydrodynamic environment have been used to provide a favorable growth environment for recombinant-adeno-associated virus vector-infected Sox9 human BMSCs. Use of this viral vector promoted the differentiation of these BMSCs into chondrocytes, potentially yielding therapeutic efficacy.[76] Other authors have transplanted transfected BMSCs into osteochondral defects in animal models and have demonstrated improvements in cartilage repair. Leng and colleagues applied calcium alginate gels mixed with BMSCs transfected with hIGF-1 cDNA into osteochondral defects on goat femoral condylar defects using mosaicplasty techniques. These authors showed improved scores on quantitative histologic assessment in the animals treated with the augmented BMSCs. Although genetically modified MSCs hold great potential in the treatment of osteochondral lesions, their safety profile has not been determined in humans, and further research is needed before augmented MSCs will be widely available for clinical application.

CLINICS CARE POINTS

- Although many orthobiologics demonstrate promise in the treatment of various foot and ankle pathologic conditions, practitioners must be aware that many claims remain without substantial evidential basis and must caution their patients appropriately.

- Bone marrow stimulation techniques for chondral injuries are generally effective but evidence is mixed throughout the literature. Surgeons should carefully evaluate the literature before choosing adjunctive techniques or additives geared toward the enhancement of stimulation procedures.

- There remains no clear superiority of one particular scaffold for orthobiologic delivery but practitioners should remain vigilant and abreast of the literature as new research is published in this area.

SUMMARY

In summary, the last several decades have brought about substantial development in our understanding of the biomolecular pathways associated with chondral disease and progression to arthritis and have provided translational investigators with many potential avenues for amelioration. Because novel therapeutics in viral-vector–mediated genetic augmentation of harvested MSCs and ACI and improvements in scaffolding materials and exogenous marrow stimulation compounds continue to be explored in animal models, widely available arthritis-retarding therapies for use in humans may greatly influence orthopedic medicine in the future.

DISCLOSURE

None.

REFERENCES

1. Sophia Fox AJ, Bedi A, Rodeo SA. The basic science of articular cartilage: structure, composition, and function. Sports health 2009;1(6):461–8.
2. D'Lima DD, Hashimoto S, Chen PC, et al. Human chondrocyte apoptosis in response to mechanical injury. Osteoarthritis Cartilage 2001;9(8):712–9.
3. Lindsjo J. Operative treatment of ankle fractures. Acta Orthop Scand Suppl 1981; 189:1–131.
4. Kraeutler M, Kaenkumchorn T, Pascual-Garrido C, et al. Peculiarities in ankle cartilage. Cartilage 2017;8:12–8.
5. Adams S, Setton L, Bell R, et al. Inflammatory cytokines and matrix metalloproteinases in the synovial fluid after intra-articular ankle fracture. Foot Ankle Int 2015; 36:1264–71.
6. Adams SB, Setton LA, Bell RD, et al. Inflammatory Cytokines and Matrix Metalloproteinases in the Synovial Fluid After Intra-articular Ankle Fracture. Foot Ankle Int 2015;36(11):1264–71.
7. Szwedowski D, Szczepanek J, Ł Paczesny, et al. Genetics in Cartilage Lesions: Basic Science and Therapy Approaches. Int J Mol Sci 2020;21(15). https://doi.org/10.3390/ijms21155430.
8. Yang C-Y, Chanalaris A, Troeberg L. ADAMTS and ADAM metalloproteinases in osteoarthritis–looking beyond the 'usual suspects'. Osteoarthritis Cartilage 2017;25(7):1000–9.
9. Rose BJ, Kooyman DL. A tale of two joints: the role of matrix metalloproteases in cartilage biology. Dis Markers 2016;2016.
10. Murphy G, Lee M. What are the roles of metalloproteinases in cartilage and bone damage? Ann Rheum Dis 2005;64(suppl 4):iv44–7.
11. Liacini A, Sylvester J, Li WQ, et al. Induction of matrix metalloproteinase-13 gene expression by TNF-α is mediated by MAP kinases, AP-1, and NF-κB transcription factors in articular chondrocytes. Exp Cell Res 2003;288(1):208–17.
12. Burrage PS, Mix KS, Brinckerhoff CE. Matrix metalloproteinases: role in arthritis. Frontiers in Bioscience-Landmark 2006;11(1):529–43.
13. Adams SB, Reilly RM, Huebner JL, et al. Time-Dependent Effects on Synovial Fluid Composition During the Acute Phase of Human Intra-articular Ankle Fracture. Foot Ankle Int 2017;38(10):1055–63.
14. Wahl EP, Lampley AJ, Chen A, et al. Inflammatory cytokines and matrix metalloproteinases in the synovial fluid after intra-articular elbow fracture. J Shoulder Elbow Surg 2020;29(4):736–42.
15. Adams SB, Leimer EM, Setton LA, et al. Inflammatory Microenvironment Persists After Bone Healing in Intra-articular Ankle Fractures. Foot Ankle Int 2017;38(5): 479–84.
16. Knäuper V, López-Otin C, Smith B, et al. Biochemical characterization of human collagenase-3. J Biol Chem 1996;271(3):1544–50.
17. Manka SW, Carafoli F, Visse R, et al. Structural insights into triple-helical collagen cleavage by matrix metalloproteinase 1. Proc Natl Acad Sci USA 2012;109(31): 12461–6.
18. Bertini I, Calderone V, Cerofolini L, et al. The catalytic domain of MMP-1 studied through tagged lanthanides. FEBS (Fed Eur Biochem Soc) Lett 2012;586(5): 557–67.
19. Knäuper V, Will H, López-Otin C, et al. Cellular mechanisms for human procollagenase-3 (MMP-13) activation: evidence that MT1-MMP (MMP-14) and

gelatinase A (MMP-2) are able to generate active enzyme. J Biol Chem 1996; 271(29):17124–31.

20. Knäuper V, Bailey L, Worley JR, et al. Cellular activation of proMMP-13 by MT1-MMP depends on the C-terminal domain of MMP-13. FEBS (Fed Eur Biochem Soc) Lett 2002;532(1–2):127–30.

21. Jackson MT, Moradi B, Smith MM, et al. Activation of matrix metalloproteinases 2, 9, and 13 by activated protein C in human osteoarthritic cartilage chondrocytes. Arthritis Rheumatol 2014;66(6):1525–36.

22. Murphy G. Tissue inhibitors of metalloproteinases. Genome Biol 2011;12:1–7.

23. Sahebjam S, Khokha R, Mort JS. Increased collagen and aggrecan degradation with age in the joints of Timp3−/− mice. Arthritis Rheum 2007;56(3):905–9.

24. Lim NH, Kashiwagi M, Visse R, et al. Reactive-site mutants of N-TIMP-3 that selectively inhibit ADAMTS-4 and ADAMTS-5: biological and structural implications. Biochem J 2010;431(1):113–22.

25. Fortier LA, Barker JU, Strauss EJ, et al. The role of growth factors in cartilage repair. Clin Orthop Relat Res 2011;469:2706–15.

26. Niu S, Anastasio AT, Faraj RR, et al. Evaluation of Heterotopic Ossification After Using Recombinant Human Bone Morphogenetic Protein-2 in Transforaminal Lumbar Interbody Fusion: A Computed Tomography Review of 996 Disc Levels. Global Spine J 2020;10(3):280–5.

27. Anastasio AT, Zinger BS, Anastasio TJ. A Novel Application of Neural Networks to Identify Potentially Effective Combinations of Biologic Factors for Enhancement of Bone Fusion/Repair. PLoS One 2022;. https://journals.plos.org/plosone/article?id=10.1371/journal.pone.0276562.

28. Tuan RS, Chen AF, Klatt BA. Cartilage regeneration. J Am Acad Orthop Surg 2013;21(5):303.

29. Sawaji Y, Hynes J, Vincent T, et al. Fibroblast growth factor 2 inhibits induction of aggrecanase activity in human articular cartilage. Arthritis Rheum 2008;58(11):3498–509.

30. Chia SL, Sawaji Y, Burleigh A, et al. Fibroblast growth factor 2 is an intrinsic chondroprotective agent that suppresses ADAMTS-5 and delays cartilage degradation in murine osteoarthritis. Arthritis Rheum 2009;60(7):2019–27.

31. Fortier LA, Balkman CE, Sandell LJ, et al. Insulin-like growth factor-I gene expression patterns during spontaneous repair of acute articular cartilage injury. J Orthop Res 2001;19(4):720–8.

32. Ricciotti E, FitzGerald GA. Prostaglandins and inflammation. Arterioscler Thromb Vasc Biol 2011;31(5):986–1000.

33. Scanzello CR, McKeon B, Swaim BH, et al. Synovial inflammation in patients undergoing arthroscopic meniscectomy: molecular characterization and relationship to symptoms. Arthritis Rheum 2011;63(2):391–400.

34. Mobasheri A, Henrotin Y, Biesalski H-K, et al. Scientific evidence and rationale for the development of curcumin and resveratrol as nutraceutricals for joint health. Int J Mol Sci 2012;13(4):4202–32.

35. Tong Z, Liu Y, Chen B, et al. Association between MMP3 and TIMP3 polymorphisms and risk of osteoarthritis. Oncotarget 2017;8(48):83563.

36. Wang T, Liang Y, Li H, et al. Single nucleotide polymorphisms and osteoarthritis: an overview and a meta-analysis. Medicine 2016;95(7).

37. Guo W, Xu P, Jin T, et al. MMP-3 gene polymorphisms are associated with increased risk of osteoarthritis in Chinese men. Oncotarget 2017;8(45):79491.

38. Southam L, Rodriguez-Lopez J, Wilkins JM, et al. An SNP in the 5′-UTR of GDF5 is associated with osteoarthritis susceptibility in Europeans and with in vivo

differences in allelic expression in articular cartilage. Hum Mol Genet 2007; 16(18):2226–32.

39. Parrish WR, Byers BA, Su D, et al. Intra-articular therapy with recombinant human GDF5 arrests disease progression and stimulates cartilage repair in the rat medial meniscus transection (MMT) model of osteoarthritis. Osteoarthritis Cartilage 2017;25(4):554–60.

40. Szczepanek J. Role of microRNA dysregulation in childhood acute leukemias: Diagnostics, monitoring and therapeutics: A comprehensive review. World J Clin Oncol 2020;11(6):348.

41. Endisha H, Rockel J, Jurisica I, et al. The complex landscape of microRNAs in articular cartilage: biology, pathology, and therapeutic targets. JCI insight 2018;3(17).

42. Wang H, Zhang H, Sun Q, et al. Intra-articular delivery of antago-miR-483-5p inhibits osteoarthritis by modulating matrilin 3 and tissue inhibitor of metalloproteinase 2. Mol Ther 2017;25(3):715–27.

43. Ko J-Y, Lee MS, Lian W-S, et al. MicroRNA-29a counteracts synovitis in knee osteoarthritis pathogenesis by targeting VEGF. Sci Rep 2017;7(1):1–14.

44. Anastasio AT, Paniagua A, Diamond C, et al. Nanomaterial Nitric Oxide Delivery in Traumatic Orthopedic Regenerative Medicine. Review. Front Bioeng Biotechnol 2021;8. https://doi.org/10.3389/fbioe.2020.592008.

45. Ramponi L, Yasui Y, Murawski CD, et al. Lesion Size Is a Predictor of Clinical Outcomes After Bone Marrow Stimulation for Osteochondral Lesions of the Talus: A Systematic Review. Am J Sports Med 2017;45(7):1698–705.

46. Yasui Y, Ramponi L, Seow D, et al. Systematic review of bone marrow stimulation for osteochondral lesion of talus - evaluation for level and quality of clinical studies. World J Orthop 2017;8(12):956–63.

47. Toale J, Shimozono Y, Mulvin C, et al. Midterm Outcomes of Bone Marrow Stimulation for Primary Osteochondral Lesions of the Talus: A Systematic Review. Orthop J Sports Med 2019;7(10). https://doi.org/10.1177/2325967119879127. 2325967119879127.

48. Park JH, Park KH, Cho JY, et al. Bone Marrow Stimulation for Osteochondral Lesions of the Talus: Are Clinical Outcomes Maintained 10 Years Later? Am J Sports Med 2021;49(5):1220–6.

49. Rikken QGH, Dahmen J, Reilingh ML, et al. Outcomes of Bone Marrow Stimulation for Secondary Osteochondral Lesions of the Talus Equal Outcomes for Primary Lesions. Cartilage 2021;13(1_suppl):1429S–37S.

50. Ivkovic A, Pascher A, Hudetz D, et al. Articular cartilage repair by genetically modified bone marrow aspirate in sheep. Gene Ther 2010;17(6):779–89.

51. Cucchiarini M, Madry H. Overexpression of human IGF-I via direct rAAV-mediated gene transfer improves the early repair of articular cartilage defects in vivo. Gene Ther 2014;21(9):811–9.

52. Cucchiarini M, Madry H, Ma C, et al. Improved tissue repair in articular cartilage defects in vivo by rAAV-mediated overexpression of human fibroblast growth factor 2. Mol Ther 2005;12(2):229–38.

53. Pascher A, Palmer G, Steinert A, et al. Gene delivery to cartilage defects using coagulated bone marrow aspirate. Gene Ther 2004;11(2):133–41.

54. Sieker J, Kunz M, Weissenberger M, et al. Direct bone morphogenetic protein 2 and Indian hedgehog gene transfer for articular cartilage repair using bone marrow coagulates. Osteoarthritis Cartilage 2015;23(3):433–42.

55. Murphy EP, McGoldrick NP, Curtin M, et al. A prospective evaluation of bone marrow aspirate concentrate and microfracture in the treatment of osteochondral lesions of the talus. Foot Ankle Surg 2019;25(4):441–8.

56. Boffa A, Previtali D, Altamura SA, et al. Platelet-Rich Plasma Augmentation to Microfracture Provides a Limited Benefit for the Treatment of Cartilage Lesions: A Meta-analysis. Orthop J Sports Med 2020;8(4). https://doi.org/10.1177/2325967120910504. 2325967120910504.

57. Schneider TE, Karaikudi S. Matrix-Induced Autologous Chondrocyte Implantation (MACI) grafting for osteochondral lesions of the talus. Foot Ankle Int 2009;30(9):810–4.

58. Ventura A, Memeo A, Borgo E, et al. Repair of osteochondral lesions in the knee by chondrocyte implantation using the MACI(R) technique. Knee Surg Sports Traumatol Arthrosc 2012;20(1):121–6.

59. Dekker TJ, Erickson B, Adams SB, et al. Topical Review: MACI as an Emerging Technology for the Treatment of Talar Osteochondral Lesions. Foot Ankle Int 2017;38(9):1045–8.

60. Lenz CG, Tan S, Carey AL, et al. Matrix-Induced Autologous Chondrocyte Implantation (MACI) Grafting for Osteochondral Lesions of the Talus. Foot Ankle Int 2020;41(9):1099–105.

61. Richter M, Zech S, Meissner S, et al. Autologous matrix induced chondrogenesis plus peripheral blood concentrate (AMIC+PBC) in chondral lesions at the ankle as part of a complex surgical approach - 5-year follow-up. Foot Ankle Surg 2022;28(8):1321–6.

62. Orth P, Kaul G, Cucchiarini M, et al. Transplanted articular chondrocytes co-overexpressing IGF-I and FGF-2 stimulate cartilage repair in vivo. Knee Surg Sports Traumatol Arthrosc 2011;19:2119–30.

63. Kang R, Marui T, Ghivizzani SC, et al. Ex vivo gene transfer to chondrocytes in full-thickness articular cartilage defects: a feasibility study. Osteoarthritis Cartilage 1997;5(2):139–43.

64. Ortved KF, Begum L, Mohammed HO, et al. Implantation of rAAV5-IGF-I transduced autologous chondrocytes improves cartilage repair in full-thickness defects in the equine model. Mol Ther 2015;23(2):363–73.

65. Ha C-W, Noh MJ, Choi KB, et al. Initial phase I safety of retrovirally transduced human chondrocytes expressing transforming growth factor-beta-1 in degenerative arthritis patients. Cytotherapy 2012;14(2):247–56.

66. Evans C, Liu F-J, Glatt V, et al. Use of genetically modified muscle and fat grafts to repair defects in bone and cartilage. Eur Cell Mater 2009;18:96.

67. Rowland CR, Glass KA, Ettyreddy AR, et al. Regulation of decellularized tissue remodeling via scaffold-mediated lentiviral delivery in anatomically-shaped osteochondral constructs. Biomaterials 2018;177:161–75.

68. Cucchiarini M, Madry H. Biomaterial-guided delivery of gene vectors for targeted articular cartilage repair. Nat Rev Rheumatol 2019;15(1):18–29.

69. Rey-Rico A, Venkatesan JK, Frisch J, et al. Effective and durable genetic modification of human mesenchymal stem cells via controlled release of rAAV vectors from self-assembling peptide hydrogels with a maintained differentiation potency. Acta Biomater 2015;18:118–27.

70. Rey-Rico A, Venkatesan JK, Schmitt G, et al. Effective remodelling of human osteoarthritic cartilage by sox9 gene transfer and overexpression upon delivery of rAAV vectors in polymeric micelles. Mol Pharm 2018;15(7):2816–26.

71. Rey-Rico A, Babicz H, Madry H, et al. Supramolecular polypseudorotaxane gels for controlled delivery of rAAV vectors in human mesenchymal stem cells for regenerative medicine. Int J Pharm 2017;531(2):492–503.
72. Brunger JM, Huynh NP, Guenther CM, et al. Scaffold-mediated lentiviral transduction for functional tissue engineering of cartilage. Proc Natl Acad Sci USA 2014;111(9):E798–806.
73. Anastasio A, Gergues M, Lebhar MS, et al. Isolation and characterization of mesenchymal stem cells in orthopaedics and the emergence of compact bone mesenchymal stem cells as a promising surgical adjunct. World J Stem Cells 2020;12(11):1341–53.
74. Freitag J, Wickham J, Shah K, et al. Effect of autologous adipose-derived mesenchymal stem cell therapy in the treatment of an osteochondral lesion of the ankle. BMJ Case Rep 2020;13(7). https://doi.org/10.1136/bcr-2020-234595.
75. Chimutengwende-Gordon M, Ahmad MA, Bentley G, et al. Stem cell transplantation for the treatment of osteochondral defects of the knee: Operative technique for a single-stage transplantation procedure using bone marrow-derived mesenchymal stem cells. Knee 2021;28:400–9.
76. Venkatesan JK, Gardner O, Rey-Rico A, et al. Improved chondrogenic differentiation of rAAV SOX9-modified human MSCs seeded in fibrin-polyurethane scaffolds in a hydrodynamic environment. Int J Mol Sci 2018;19(9):2635.

Moving?

Make sure your subscription moves with you!

To notify us of your new address, find your **Clinics Account Number** (located on your mailing label above your name), and contact customer service at:

Email: journalscustomerservice-usa@elsevier.com

800-654-2452 (subscribers in the U.S. & Canada)
314-447-8871 (subscribers outside of the U.S. & Canada)

Fax number: 314-447-8029

Elsevier Health Sciences Division
Subscription Customer Service
3251 Riverport Lane
Maryland Heights, MO 63043

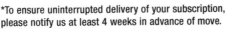

Printed and bound by CPI Group (UK) Ltd, Croydon, CR0 4YY

08/05/2025

01864748-0010